AFTER THE WAR

AFTER
THE WAR

Surviving PTSD and Changing Mental Health Culture

STÉPHANE GRENIER

with Adam Montgomery

 University of Regina Press

Printed and bound in Canada at Marquis. The text of this book is printed on 100% post-consumer recycled paper with earth-friendly vegetable-based inks.

Cover and text design: Duncan Campbell, University of Regina Press
Copy editor: Ryan Perks
Proofreader: Kristine Douaud
Indexer: Sergey Lobachev, Brookfield Indexing Services
Cover art: Portrait of Stéphane Grenier by Philip Cheung, www.philipcheungphoto.com.

Library and Archives Canada Cataloguing in Publication

Grenier, Stéphane, 1965-, author

After the war : surviving PTSD and changing mental health culture / Stéphane Grenier with Adam Montgomery.

Includes bibliographical references and index.
Issued in print and electronic formats. ISBN 978-0-88977-533-6 (softcover).—
ISBN 978-0-88977-534-3 (PDF).—ISBN 978-0-88977-535-0 (HTML)

1. Grenier, Stéphane, 1965- —Mental health. 2. Grenier, Stéphane, 1965-. 3. Soldiers—Mental health—Canada. 4. Soldiers—Mental health services—Canada. 5. Veterans—Mental health—Canada. 6. Veterans—Mental health services—Canada. 7. Traumatic neuroses. 8. Mental health services—Canada. 9. Mental health promotion—Canada. I. Montgomery, Adam, 1982-, author II. Title.

RC552.P67G74 2018   616.85′210092   C2017-906786-9   C2017-906787-7

10 9 8 7 6 5 4 3 2 1

University of Regina Press, University of Regina
Regina, Saskatchewan, Canada, S4S 0A2
TEL: (306) 585-4758 FAX: (306) 585-4699
U OF R PRESS   WEB: www.uofrpress.ca

We acknowledge the support of the Canada Council for the Arts for our publishing program. We acknowledge the financial support of the Government of Canada. / Nous reconnaissons l'appui financier du gouvernement du Canada. This publication was made possible with support from Creative Saskatchewan's Creative Industries Production Grant Program.

Canada Council   Conseil des arts
for the Arts   du Canada

Canadä

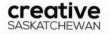

CONTENTS

ACKNOWLEDGEMENTS

I wish to start by expressing my gratitude to my family. A special and heartfelt thanks first and foremost to Julie, my partner and strongest supporter for over three decades. My son, David, and my daughter, Véronique, gave me the strength to carry on when I was at my lowest. I have been so proud to watch them grow up and become great Canadians. My granddaughter, Zora, occupies a special place in my heart, and represents for me the generation that I hope will enjoy the fruits of our hard work transforming the mental health system.

From my time in the Canadian Armed Forces I want to thank John Blouin for the long days, dedication, and friendship he gave me during and after our time in Rwanda. David Snashall was a great friend and his *joie de vivre* inspired me on many missions abroad. Joel Brayman deserves special thanks for being the first to recognize that I wasn't well after my return from Rwanda. Michel Arsenault was my first peer supporter, and he gave me the perspective I needed to get help. Thanks to Chris Corrigan for his unconditional support as my commander in Toronto. Chris was a stellar leader and friend, and his empathy allowed me to start on my path to recovery. Christian Couture, may he rest in peace, provided me with the soil to sow the seeds of peer support in the Canadian military, and I will be forever grateful for his kind, compassionate leadership. Rick Noseworthy excelled as the first OSISS peer supporter and was also a great friend throughout my career, and beyond. Thanks to Marc Godfrey for keeping both me and my staff grounded during our formative years delivering peer support to the military.

Christian McEachern was a great sounding board; he deserves many thanks for being the soldier who made me realize just how much peer support was needed in the Canadian Forces. David Wrather was a great boss and leader as I created OSISS; he took a big risk trusting in our vision. Thanks, David. Dr. Don Richardson was the first psychiatrist to believe in my idea and in the OSISS program, and he has been a trusted friend and colleague ever since. I must also mention Jim Woodley, whom I pulled out of retirement to be my right-hand man in managing the program. Kathy Darte of Veterans Affairs Canada was a voice of reason, someone who worked hard to create acceptance of my non-clinical vision. Jim Jamieson's tireless efforts helped us convince clinicians at the Department of National Defence that peer support was beneficial for their patients. Sophie Richard worked, and still works, tirelessly with military families, and she helped me to expand the OSISS program to those who also carry the consequences of military service. Marianne LeBeau kept the program rooted for many years, and helped OSISS stay within its founding mission. Lastly, I wish to extend my thanks to the entire OSISS team—past, present, and future. Your important work has changed so many lives for the better. You are all true heroes.

A quick word of thanks to my former colleagues on the Mental Health Commission of Canada's Workforce Advisory Committee. They supported my vision of peer support, and I am very grateful for that.

I also wish to acknowledge my friends and colleagues at Peer Support Accreditation and Certification Canada, as well as those in the civilian mental health sphere. I am thankful to Dr. Ian Arnold for all his hard work and friendship, and for his helpful insights and commentary during the production of this book. Dr. Rachel Thibault has been a tireless worker in the cause of peer support, and I am blessed to have her as a colleague. Annette and Vital Ducharme have given countless volunteer hours to the cause. Dr. Jayne Barker was a supporter and believer in our work, and she went to bat for us as we pushed peer support beyond its former boundaries within the Mental

Health Commission. Thanks to the late Diana Capponi and all the other peer supporters across Canada who allowed me to better understand the challenges faced by ordinary Canadians trying to access the mental health system. Thanks also to the past, present, and future board members of PSACC for their tireless dedication to starting and sustaining a new charitable organization. My most heartfelt thanks go to Kim Sunderland for taking on the daunting challenge of being our first executive director. Shaleen Jones also deserves mention for accepting to lead our charity through some difficult times.

Sincere thanks also go out to my colleagues at Mental Health Innovations, Kim Sunderland, Marie-Josée Michaud, Leslie Bennett, and Jon O'Connor, who are great innovators. I am also very grateful to Richard Dixon and Lyne Wilson, at NAV Canada, for giving myself and MHI its first big break, and for understanding how peer support can enhance Canadian workplaces. Special thanks to Dr. Linda Courey and the Nova Scotia Health Authority for committing to community peer support at the provincial level. Thanks also to Lauren Scott for accepting the challenge of managing a complex program, and to our present and future peer supporters.

I also wish to acknowledge those on my journey who stigmatized people undergoing mental health challenges. This includes those who felt the status quo was sufficient, and who told me that I wasn't capable enough or didn't have the appropriate academic credentials to influence change. I say this without a hint of acrimony, because if it hadn't been for those people the need for change may not have been as obvious to me.

And finally, I want to acknowledge a young man who helped make this book a reality. Adam Montgomery and I met a few years ago while he was finishing his PhD. When I read his dissertation, in which he so masterfully captured the reality that soldiers face after overseas service, I knew that he was the right fit to help me write this book. His first book, *The Invisible Injured*, is a must-read, and a kind of companion to *After the War* for those who want to dig deeper.

For anyone else whose name I have unintentionally missed, my apologies.

PREFACE

Writing this story with my co-author Adam Montgomery, I encountered a few difficulties common to anyone who attempts to fit together the pieces of a story that occurred in the distant past—in some cases over twenty years ago. The first had to do with the vagaries of long-term memory and the way in which names, dates, and events can become blurred with the passage of time. The second, more personal difficulty related to the mental injuries that I sustained during my 1994–95 peacekeeping tour in Rwanda. Memories of that experience, as well as my troubles afterward, are still vivid, but in some cases their chronological order is difficult to sort out. To mitigate any factual errors and misattributions, Adam and I have done our best to triangulate events, names, and dates by using contemporary journalistic accounts, consulting literature on both the Rwandan genocide and mental health, and relying on the memory of others involved in the stories related here. I hope that you, the reader, will forgive any errors that may have slipped through the cracks.

You should also be forewarned that the following pages contain some very graphic and emotionally disturbing scenes, particularly those relating to my tour in Rwanda. I feel it's necessary to relate these stories, however troubling, to show how my memories of these events have shaped my life. In particular, I want you to see how I used them to find solutions for my own mental health challenges, to improve the military's approach to mental health, and to illuminate the burgeoning mental health problem in Canadian society. I must note in closing that some names have been changed to preserve the privacy of the individuals involved.

ABBREVIATIONS

DND   Department of National Defence
EAP   Employee Assistance Program
LAV   Light Armoured Vehicle
LFCAHQ   Land Force Central Area Headquarters
MHCC   Mental Health Commission of Canada
MHI   Mental Health Innovations
MLO   Media Liaison Office
NDHQ   National Defence Headquarters
NDMC   National Defence Medical Centre
NIS   National Investigation Service
OSI   operational stress injury
OSISS   Operational Stress Injury Social Support program
PSACC   Peer Support Accreditation and Certification Canada
RGF   Rwandan Government Forces
RPA   Rwandan Patriotic Army
RPF   Rwandan Patriotic Front
TLD   third location decompression
UNHQ   United Nations Headquarters (Kigali)

Chapter 1

INTO THE KILLING FIELDS

R wanda, early May 1994. Torrential rain was falling as the CC-130 Hercules transport plane landed at Kigali International Airport. Here, in this small African country, a civil war raged. The second phase of this war had begun less than a month earlier, but the warring factions—the Rwandan Government Forces (RGF) and the Rwandan Patriotic Front (RPF)—had lately been obeying a temporary ceasefire, allowing our transport to land and deliver humanitarian aid.* Rwanda is a land-locked country, and during the war the airport was the only straightforward way in or out; this made it a vital landmark for military strategists. Ours was the only aircraft in the world cleared to land there that day.

On board were some basic supplies and several peacekeepers—myself included—sent to bolster an overstretched and beleaguered UN force. But as the plane touched down it became apparent to everyone on board that the combatants had decided to carry on fighting regardless of the ceasefire, and tracer rounds could be seen darting

---

* The RGF were also known as the Rwandan Armed Forces, or, in French, the Forces armées rwandaises.

through the air all around us.* The gunfire made the pilot quite nervous, and he decided to leave the engines running to ease his escape. His main concern, after dropping us off and unloading the plane's cargo, was to get out of there as quickly as possible—and who could blame him? Within a few minutes our equipment was on the tarmac. Several pallets of six-by-six wooden beams and corrugated steel roofing panels had also been unloaded by a diesel-engine forklift spewing black smoke into the air. As it chugged along, Kigali's natural odours mixed with diesel fuel and invaded my nostrils—a smell that would be forever seared in my brain.

We were quickly ushered by UN peacekeepers behind a few pallets, where we were to await our transport to UN Headquarters, or UNHQ, as we came to call it. After a few minutes passed, the CC-130's engines roared. The plane began to roll away, gradually accelerating onto the runway, where it picked up speed and lifted off. As the plane's humming engine faded into the distance the cracking sound of gunfire once again emerged to take its place. War-torn Rwanda: this would be my new home, my new workplace, my new reality for the next ten months.

Some fellow peacekeepers divided us into various vehicles for the short trip to UNHQ, which was at the Amahoro Stadium Hotel, a building located beside Rwanda's largest sports stadium. The stadium and hotel were about halfway between the airport and downtown Kigali, and they had been taken over by the UN mission's Canadian commander, Major-General Roméo Dallaire. Of course, the complex's designation as a UN-protected site didn't stop the warring factions from occasionally firing on or attempting to enter it.

On our trip from the airport I sat in the front passenger seat of a beat-up Land Rover. I introduced myself to the Canadian soldier driving it, but he was uninterested in pleasantries, and gave me only a brief

---

*   Traditionally, every fifth round in a machine gun ammunition belt is loaded with a small pyrotechnic charge, which causes the round to burn brightly when fired, even during the day. Tracer rounds allow the gunner to "trace" where his rounds are hitting, and to correct fire accordingly.

nod. His thoughts seemed to be focused solely on getting us—and himself—to the relative safety of UNHQ. In spite of the pouring rain and the high humidity, the vehicle's defogger and windshield wipers were both inoperative, which meant we had almost no visibility. The driver drove way too fast, now and then barely steering around the craters left by incoming mortar rounds. At one point he hit the brakes and skidded around an object; as we went by I caught a glimpse of an unexploded mortar bomb sticking halfway out of the asphalt. I wondered what driving over one of those would do. I was lucky that I never found out.

The windshield fogged over, I began scanning the terrain through the passenger window. One of the first things I noticed was how rich the Rwandan soil was; it was a beautiful red I hadn't seen anywhere in Canada. The next thing that caught my eye was a woman in the distance, squatting and relieving herself. Then, a little ways down the road, without warning, I saw my first human corpse. Because of the weather conditions and time of day I couldn't tell for sure if it was a man or a woman: they just lay there by the side of the road, like a piece of unwanted garbage someone had pitched from their vehicle. The limbs looked dislocated and mangled, and it was obvious the person had met a sudden, violent death. This was the first of thousands of corpses I would see during my tour of Rwanda.

Of course, I had seen dead people before. Like most adults I had been to a funeral, and had seen war movies and documentaries about the Holocaust. But seeing actual bodies in a conflict setting made the shock of death hit home in an eerily visceral way. The soil's redness was now associated in my mind with blood, which imparted its own shade of red all over the ground. Indeed, that first mangled body was soon followed by several others as we drove to UNHQ. Doing my best to remain stoic, I thought to myself, "Don't be surprised, you saw the news and heard the stories." And yet nothing could prepare me for the actual event. Along with the rain, the bullets, and the generalized chaos swirling around me, these surreal scenes of death amounted to a sort of "Welcome to Rwanda" message. I was unaware that the mission I was then embarking on would change my life forever.

When we first arrived at UNHQ there were no sleeping quarters left, so I was brought to a hotel owned by the Belgian airline Sabena. Unfortunately, by that point the hotel was a refugee camp. Armed UN soldiers from Ghana guarded the entrance, and the walls were riddled with bullet holes from the fighting that had raged there in the weeks before my arrival. The lobby was quite large and because of its lack of lighting had the feel of a dark cave. I could smell wood coals burning, and somewhere off in the darkness I could hear the cries and moans of someone in pain. After climbing a large staircase my team eventually entered an unoccupied room. It was about 150 square feet in size and smelled like a mixture of stale food and death. Save for some retro shag carpeting and a broken side table lying in pieces on the floor, the room was devoid of any amenities, and like the rest of the hotel it had no electricity or running water. When I entered the bathroom the first thing I saw was several dead rats scattered around the floor and along the counter. That explained some of the smell, at least. It was an unsettling place to start my tour, but it was all there was for the moment. Exhausted, we settled in for the night.

As the day drew to a close we could see more tracer rounds fly over Kigali. From what I could tell the combatants wanted to get off their last shots before nighttime arrived. (They didn't have sophisticated weaponry or night-vision devices, so combat usually stopped when darkness came, offering a period of relative calm.) I noticed a series of trenches off in the distance, but I never did figure out which side had made them because the front line kept moving according to the changing military situation. That night I ate a German army ration containing some sort of pâté and crackers. It wasn't the tastiest meal, but it was nutritious, and under the circumstances I was happy to eat anything at all. My journey had taken me by military bus from Ottawa to Canadian Forces Base Trenton, where I caught a military plane to Nairobi, Kenya. From there I boarded the CC-130 that took me to Kigali. The total travel time was almost two days. Physically exhausted, I was more than ready to sleep; the difficult part, I soon realized, was trying to clear my head of what I'd seen during the day.

My work as a UN peacekeeper would soon take me across many different regions of Rwanda. Early in my deployment I was part of a team that visited a Rwandan Patriotic Army (RPA) training camp. The RPA was the Tutsi-dominated military wing of the RPF, a rebel group comprised of Rwandan refugees, many of whom had been raised in Ugandan refugee camps. Controlled by Paul Kagame, the current (as of 2017) Rwandan president, the RPA was by 1994 attempting to wrestle control of the country from the Hutu-dominated RGF. The UN's task was to help build trusting relations between the warring factions—a difficult task at the best of times, given the complete distrust and animosity they felt for one another. We had intended our unscheduled visit to the RPA camp as a sort of impromptu spot check, to remind them of the UN's presence and gently push them away from combat operations.

As we drove into the camp an eerie atmosphere seemed to pervade the whole area. There was not a single person in sight, and the only sign of movement came from the grass as it swayed in a gentle breeze. The camp was built on a sloped hill with a main road that took us up to the compound. When we reached the top we parked and got out to look around. We walked to the side of the hill, looked down at the next plateau below, and saw a bicycle on its side. The back wheel, parallel to the ground, was slowly turning, as if someone from a film crew had spun the wheel and moved out of the way and yelled "ACTION!" We all stood in silence, wondering what was going on. But things slowly came into focus, and we noticed shapes and forms on either side of the bike. Then, we saw clothing. Finally, hands and feet became visible: more dead bodies.

We made our way down the hill to see if there were any survivors. As we approached, it became obvious that the bodies, which were quite bloated, had been there for some time. Investigating further, we began to discover other corpses as well. I was unaccustomed to seeing dead bodies, yet here they seemed to just pop out of nowhere. There were a series of small buildings around the plateau, some with doors still shut and others wide open. In one building we found a pile of men stacked on top of one another, like sacks of rice in a warehouse.

Judging from their state of decomposition they had been dead for a few days. A couple of minutes later we walked into a larger building, searching for any signs of life. As I walked around inside I turned and was suddenly startled by a large Ghanaian soldier from our team; he was standing directly behind me, holding a machete at eye level and examining the blade. It was encrusted with rust and dried blood: we had found one of the murder weapons.

A little while later we were shocked to hear the sound of a baby crying. Hoping to find even a single survivor, something to make us feel useful, we ran towards the sound. But as we approached we realized the baby was actually a goat crying its last few breaths. Those responsible for the mass murder surrounding us felt it necessary to kill even the animals. To this day I still wonder if it was indeed the sound of a baby. On some level we needed it to be; we felt totally powerless to prevent the death and destruction all around us. I would later relive that helpless feeling whenever memories of this incident appeared in my mind.

On our way back from the deserted RPA camp the entire team was silent. This was in stark contrast to the usual banter that went on during our drives through the country. But what was the point in talking? There was nothing any of us could say to mitigate or undo the scene we had just witnessed. As we drove down the narrow dirt road we came upon a clearing, and there another tragic scene awaited us. A heavy-set man, bloated like most of the others we'd seen, lay on his back with his arms wide open. He had on a grey suit and white shirt, perhaps for a visit to church. Beside him was a little girl in a beautiful blue floral-print dress. Unlike the man—perhaps her father or grandfather—she was on her belly, with her arms tucked close to her body and her fists near her head, which was turned slightly to one side, in a posture my own young daughter often assumed while lying in bed.

I was so taken aback by the initial scene that I failed to notice the rest of its details. My first thought was of the tragedy that had struck this family. I looked around for a moment, trying to make sense of yet another horrible scene from Rwanda's unfolding genocide. For a moment I stared at the girl, following the colours of her dress from her

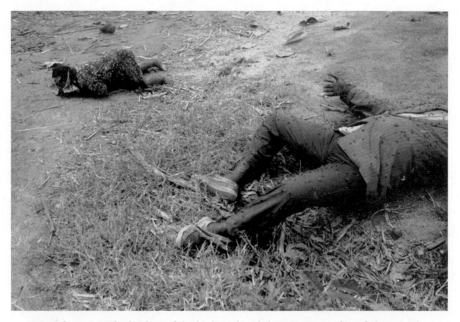

Rwanda, 1994: The bodies of the little girl and the man as we found them in the clearing.

leg to her back, but as I reached the top of her body my eyes came to an abrupt stop. One-third of her head was missing, leaving her brain exposed. Her murderers had deliberately cut her head in two pieces and left her body to rot.

ON THE RIDE back to the Amahoro Hotel my mind drifted to thoughts of my own childhood and what had led me to the point where I might witness tragedy on an unimaginable scale.

I was born in Lachute, Quebec, a small city about eighty kilometres northwest of Montreal. My mother, Jeannine Giroux, was also born in Lachute, and my father, Jean Marc Grenier, came from the Abitibi area, a predominantly French-speaking region several hundred kilometres north of Lachute that until 1868 was owned by the Hudson's Bay Company.

My father, born in April 1933, had a very humble childhood. His family was quite poor, so his options were limited. Without post-secondary education, he decided to become a construction worker. As a young man in the early 1960s he started working near a large hydroelectric plant, the Carillon Generating Station, located on the Ottawa River near Lachute. He moved to a nearby village, which is how he met my mother, who was a lot younger than my dad. She was the eldest in a family of five (four girls and one boy), and when I was a child we spent a lot of time with her parents and siblings.

Shortly after I was born my parents moved us to Montreal, where we lived in a poor area of the city. When I was five we moved to Churchill Falls, Labrador, a tiny town of several hundred people, where my father once again worked on hydroelectric projects at a generating station. Despite living in a trailer we had a happy life, but it wasn't long before we moved back to Montreal, to a community called Pierrefonds (or Bedrock, as the borough's predominately English-speaking residents would say). Eventually, when I was a teenager, my parents got divorced. There was no acrimony between them; they just decided they wanted to go their separate ways. My mom remarried three years later and had two daughters with her second husband, giving me two half-sisters, Lea and Eva.

I was a very active and gregarious kid, always playing outside and spending time with friends. In those days parents weren't afraid to let their children play outside by themselves, so I was free to escape the house from just after breakfast until dinner almost every day that I wasn't in school. I lived in anglophone surroundings in Churchill Falls, and later in Pierrefonds, so I was bilingual from a young age, speaking French at home and English outside. Most of my friends were anglophones, so I was thankfully able to maintain my bilingualism throughout my younger years despite later attending a French high school.

As a young man I was never a scholar; instead I preferred more hands-on types of activities, like fixing machines and woodworking. As for sports, I opted for football and soccer rather than hockey, and with some dedicated practise I was even able to win a few football trophies along the way. At five foot eleven, I was big for a high-school student and I was able to play the game without getting injured, but once I reached my late teens and early twenties the young men I played against were much bigger. Breaking my nose and a few fingers playing against much tougher opponents convinced me that it was time to pursue other hobbies.

I attended high school at a large Catholic boarding school in Rigaud, Quebec, a small city about halfway between Montreal and Ottawa. In the first year I was quartered in a large dormitory with numerous other students, but I was eventually given a semi-private room with one other boy; finally, in my last year, I had a room to myself. The school was a great place to come of age. I really enjoyed my time there—hanging out with the guys, playing sports, and dividing my time between studies and goofing around.

Like any other high school, mine had multiple clans. I was a part of the semi-cool, semi-sporty clan, and I was also a drummer in the school band. For some reason I was perpetually accused of smuggling drugs into the school, even though I never, ever took drugs. I think the priests in charge just didn't know what to make of me, largely because I tended to challenge authority whenever possible. If I was a disruptor, though, I believe it was in a good way.

On the first day of my final year there were several new kids at the school. One of them, Patrick, had big, thick glasses and clearly had great difficulty walking. He also couldn't hear, and so had big hearing aids hanging out of his ears. Because he'd been fitted with them relatively late in life, he had only just begun to speak at the age of fifteen. The poor guy immediately stuck out. When I saw him I walked over and welcomed him to the school. We spoke for a few minutes, and since he seemed like a nice kid I made a point of talking with him whenever I saw him after that. Most of the other kids stared at him or made quiet remarks when he walked by, but over time I tried to make myself his guardian angel of sorts. When I heard other kids had made fun of him I challenged the person who did it and told them to back off, and when I saw him eating alone I sometimes went over and joined him. Even as a selfish teenager it tore my heart out to see how the stigma of being different and people's fear of the unknown prevented other kids from being his friend (though of course I didn't understand it in such a complex, adult way back then).

During that year he turned eighteen, which in the province of Quebec means you can legally purchase alcohol. On his birthday I asked him what he wanted to do, and like most other teenagers who have reached legal age, he said he really wanted to have a beer. So later that day we went out to a local restaurant, and it made me feel good to see him smiling and enjoying himself, with partial help, no doubt, of a slight alcohol buzz. Without making too much of our friendship, looking back I can say that it was the first sense I got of how marginalized people sometimes need others to come to their aid.

I don't know whether it was nature or nurture, but my high-school years made me into a bit of a leader. Kids learned not to mess with me, and at the same time I learned that one person could make a big difference if only they had the willpower to make changes and the ability to look at the world through someone else's eyes.

My school was located on a massive property built right into a mountain, with each building occupying a different ascending level. The first and largest building was an old and massive stone structure that at its centre stood several stories high. Inside was a chapel, several classrooms, teachers' offices, dormitories for the junior students, and a gymnasium. At the other end there was an arena, sports fields, and a modern brick facility that held classrooms and senior students' bedrooms. The brick building was shaped like a capital I, with bedrooms situated at the top and down the middle, and classrooms going down from the middle to the bottom. Joining the two main buildings was an underground tunnel, designed so that students and faculty could avoid going outside during Rigaud's harsh winters. At the halfway point the tunnel also branched off toward the gymnasium, which also housed the cafeteria. During the winter, seniors would wake up, go through the tunnel to the cafeteria, and then come back to their rooms, brush their teeth, and go to class.

Since the school was run by Catholic priests, a symbol of the church's pervasive authority in Quebec in those days, the students were always looking for ways to stir things up. During the spring of my senior year, for example, there was a mass demonstration against the school cafeteria's food. Students decided that after the usual lunch period they would bring their trays outside and leave them on the hill behind the school instead of in the official washing area. Several hundred teenagers walking out with trays made quite the sight, as did the priests' attempts—all finger wagging and angry gestures—to stop them. Unsure what to do, the poor lunch ladies just stood and watched. As I looked at all the kids sitting on the hill, I couldn't help but think the whole situation was ridiculous: the food wasn't *that* bad, and the people really being hurt were the cafeteria staff, who did their best with what they had and who would now have to retrieve several hundred messy trays.

I walked up the hill to where a priest was addressing the student mob, and in a loud voice yelled out that I thought what they were doing was silly. I pointed to the cafeteria ladies standing in the distance and declared that those were the people they were really punishing—not the priest standing in front of them. After listening for a minute, a few of my fellow students directed their anger at me, but I finally convinced much of the group to abandon their demonstration. Quietly, some of the students began picking up their trays and taking them down the hill to the cafeteria. The demonstration's ringleaders walked away to another area and tried to keep fanning the flames among those still on the hill, but the majority had left. Within a half-hour everything was sorted out.

Ironically, I somehow still got in trouble. The priests didn't like that I took charge: they felt that I'd made them look bad, that I'd tried to stop the demonstration purely out of a desire for self-aggrandizement. In reality, I think they just didn't like having the appearance of power and authority taken from them, even for just a few minutes. After that they had it in for me for the rest of the year.

Looking back on my high-school years I can see now that my desire to be a leader, and to take action when I witnessed injustice, was formed in certain indelible moments like that day outside the school cafeteria. Over the years, a lot of people have asked me why I joined the military in 1983, and the most honest answer is that I really don't know for sure. But I do know that I wanted to be a part of something bigger than me, and to be part of an organization that got involved in issues and events that really meant something. I was pretty gung-ho in the early stages of my career, especially after joining the Canadian Armoured Corps, but my primary motivation was to be a part of grand events. Unfortunately, the narrative I envisioned in my head—bravely keeping the peace and making my country proud— had little to do with the horrors I witnessed eleven years later, when I was nearly thirty.

In the years after I returned from Rwanda I was sometimes unable to watch my own daughter sleep, especially when she lay in the same position as the Rwandan girl we'd encountered that day on our return from the RPA camp. One night, in fact, as I went to kiss her goodnight, I found myself frozen in the doorway. For a few seconds it was as if a candle had flickered and my daughter had been replaced by the young Rwandan girl. I stood there, paralyzed and confused, and suddenly I felt very hot and sweaty. My mind raced and I didn't know what to think or do. I remember wondering, briefly, whether or not this experience—this vision—was real. This was one of my first "flashbacks." There would be many more down the road.

A FEW DAYS after visiting the RPA camp I was standing with some civilians on the roof of the Amahoro. On it was a small bunker surrounded by sandbags. A Ghanaian peacekeeper was observing the events in Kigali through binoculars, watching troop movements and other ominous signs of civil war. The sound of gunshots in the distance kept everyone slightly on edge, and raging fires burned from several locations across the city. From the hotel roof the trouble seemed somewhat distant, but that illusion was shattered when, a few minutes later, we heard the sound of mortars somewhere behind us and saw the splashes of dirt and debris fly into the air several hundred metres away. Everyone was confused, since we didn't know who was firing on whom; the mortars seemed to be landing in the middle of nowhere. Then a mortar suddenly whistled by at close range.

It soon became clear that the hotel was in the path of destruction. I yelled to everyone that we needed to get off the roof quickly, since there wasn't enough room for us in the bunker. There were several large pipes scattered about, and a heavy-set man trying to run for cover tripped over one of them. Probably believing that he didn't have time to make it to the door, he sandwiched himself between a few of the pipes. I knew this wouldn't provide any protection, so I sprinted over, took him by the belt of his pants, and yanked him out of his hiding spot. As I threw him up on his feet he slipped and fell again, ripping his pants. Exposed in more ways than one, he now picked up his pace and ran for the door, escaping back into the relative safety of the hotel. Afterwards I checked to make sure no one else was still on the roof before following the group into the building. As soon as I got inside I heard the next mortar land slightly off in the distance. I don't know for sure whether the people firing the mortars had purposely targeted the hotel, but they had certainly got our attention—even though the entire incident happened in the space of about ten seconds. Just a typical afternoon in Rwanda.

The next day I needed to use a satellite phone to provide a situation report to the folks at National Defence Headquarters (NDHQ) in Ottawa. The phone was on the Amahoro's third-floor balcony. I was standing there, speaking with Lieutenant (Navy) Chris Henderson, when I heard a *whoosh* and felt a blast of heat close by: a rocket-propelled grenade had hit the side of the hotel, showering debris onto the balcony in front of me and throwing me to the ground. There was a slight buzzing in my ears and I felt disoriented, but after several seconds I picked up the satellite phone. All I could hear on the other end was Chris's screaming; he was unaware of what had just happened, and perhaps thought I'd been wounded or killed. But I assured him I was okay, and after a few moments we continued on with our situation report.

It was this type of surreal, unexpected event—common during my time in Rwanda—that people would later connect to my diagnosis of post-traumatic stress disorder (PTSD). But at the time I didn't really feel as though I was undergoing any "trauma." It's not that I was—or am—trying to come off like Rambo: I just didn't feel anything other than happy that I'd escaped physical injury. Psychiatrists

13

might call this event "traumatic," but even in retrospect it seems like just another day in Rwanda.

During my first week in the country, the UN launched an operation to evacuate Rwandan refugees who'd been sponsored by other countries. The war was in full swing by then, with the genocide marching in lockstep behind it. Those being evacuated were either Tutsi families or intermarried families of Tutsis and Hutus—precisely those targeted by the Interahamwe, the Hutu paramilitary organization dominated by thugs. Over the course of about a week, the UN had managed to gather all of the sponsored families at the Hôtel des Mille Collines, a place well known to anyone familiar with Roméo Dallaire's book *Shake Hands with the Devil* or the Hollywood movie *Hotel Rwanda*.

On that particular day it seemed that all of the paperwork had finally been processed, and things were moving at a good speed. By this time commercial airlines had long since stopped flying into Rwanda, but given the fact that General Dallaire, the UN commander, was Canadian, the Canadian military continued flying in CC-130s at a frequency of about two per day. Ceasefires were negotiated so that each day the planes could unload supplies, pick up people, and take off without being fired on. It was a risky arrangement at the best of times.

Dozens of trucks from various UN contingents were parked outside the hotel. The soldiers' purpose was to ensure that all refugees leaving the Mille Collines for the airport were registered and that their paperwork was in order before they were flown to Nairobi. Names were checked and identification badges given out as hundreds of refugees slowly filled the waiting UN trucks. The refugees were understandably nervous. Several weeks earlier, in April 1994, the Interahamwe had tried to use the hotel as a place to herd and murder civilians. Knowing their lives were in danger, the refugees wanted to get out of the country as quickly as possible.

Amid this sea of activity we spotted some movement in the bushes across from the parking lot. What we soon found out was that members of the Interahamwe, unhappy that these people were about to escape their grasp, were setting up a base from which to fire. Suddenly a jeep arrived, and three large men wearing an odd assortment of military camouflage and civilian clothing stepped off and looked at the crowd with a menacing glare. At first it was unclear exactly who they were, but when they started bullying refugees and UN workers, we knew they were definitely Interahamwe.

The tension quickly began to rise. Major Don MacNeil, a Canadian military observer for the UN, and head negotiator for the refugee-vetting process, confronted the thugs, telling them that we had complete clearance from both the RGF and the RPF, and that our activities were perfectly in line with our UN mandate. The militia leader was immediately upset because his threats and bullying tactics weren't working. He and his men promptly got back into their jeep and screeched out of the parking lot. Things settled down a few minutes later, and the refugee processing continued.

About ten minutes later I was walking through the parking lot when a young Rwandan boy about the same age and height as my own son walked in front of me. It was unclear, and still is to this day, whether he was an orphan or simply looking for his family. Out of nowhere, the cracking of gunfire rang out, but it was much closer than it usually was. The Interahamwe in the bushes had opened up with their machine guns, instantly turning the parking lot into a scene of screaming and chaos. Somehow, I can still remember, amid the yelling and the gunfire, the sound of one bullet in particular as it hit the boy's upper thigh. Also seared into my brain is the image of the boy being literally flipped over from the sheer power of the gun shot, like a bowling pin flying into the air and falling to the ground. The next thing I remember is me and a Rwandan man picking up the boy and rushing inside the hotel as hordes of people stampeded toward the entrance, which was shielded only by glass. The boy, evidently in immense pain, was screaming at the top of his lungs. Within less than a minute the firing stopped and the Interahamwe sped off; they had done their damage for the day. Fearing a return visit, the UN workers quickly got back to business and the evacuation of refugees began.

I rounded up my people and we headed back to UNHQ as the other teams stayed on to finish the process.

Murder and intimidation were two of the Interahamwe's principal tactics. Shortly after the incident in the Mille Collines parking lot I was with a group of Canadian reporters when we got another taste of the Interahamwe's attempts to bully and cajole UN personnel. My job was to get the reporters, who'd come to gather information about our refugee-processing efforts at the Mille Collines, safely back to UNHQ. I was in a white SUV, along with the driver and two reporters, en route to the Amahoro, which meant we had to cross several bridges that were used as checkpoints for the warring armies. One bridge had recently been captured by the Interahamwe, and orders had been given to the thugs guarding the bridge with rocket-propelled grenades, AK-47s, and machetes, to bully and harass UN peacekeepers in every possible way. When we reached the checkpoint we stopped and waited to see what would happen.

The situation was tense. Our driver was interrogated by the checkpoint commander, who attempted in the usual Interahamwe manner to obstruct us however he could, saying that we couldn't go through and that we'd have to turn around. As the discussion went on I felt someone enter my personal space: to my right a large Interahamwe soldier had poked his head and arm halfway through my window. In his hand was a machete with stains on it, and he muttered gruffly that I was a Belgian. Several weeks earlier, ten Belgian peacekeepers were brutally tortured and murdered by members of the Presidential Guard, who believed radio reports that the Belgians were responsible for assassinating Rwandan president Juvénal Habyarimana on April 6, 1994. Since Belgians were viewed as nefarious colonial masters and manipulators by many Rwandans—the country had been a Belgian colony until the early 1960s—I now worried the Interahamwe would try to kill me. The Canadian UN uniforms had a small green Canadian flag on the left shoulder, but from his side of the vehicle it wasn't visible. I told him that I was from Canada, but he kept insisting I was Belgian. I tried to show him my left shoulder, but it was difficult—it was a tight space and the man's machete was right in front of my face.

While I continued arguing with the Interahamwe soldier our driver, who was having no luck convincing the checkpoint guard to let us through, decided it was time for a drastic decision. He put his foot to the pedal, and we crashed through the checkpoint in a mad dash. Gunfire erupted behind us, and I'm sure all of us felt a cold shiver go up our spine as we anticipated being shot in the back. But we were lucky; the Interahamwe were poor soldiers and couldn't aim very well, and in the end we made it out without any injuries. But the experience left its mark on our memories nonetheless, and I had numerous dreams about the incident after my return to Canada. In each of them I was Belgian instead of Canadian. I hated those nights.

After a week and a half in Rwanda I was given the task of escorting members of the media on their flight back to Nairobi, from which they would fly home. Like most days, a ceasefire had been negotiated on May 9 to allow the Canadian Hercules to fly out of Kigali. The previous night at the Amahoro had been a harrowing one. We spent the night sleeping on the ground in a glass rotunda, and at about 4:30 a.m. we were woken by the sound of a mortar round falling dangerously close to the building. This was both a metaphorical and literal wake-up call for some, telling them it was time to get out of Rwanda. I can't recall much of what happened after I got up, but I know it was a busy day of fighting for the warring factions, which meant plenty of gunfire around the city. The drive to the airport was tense, and as we walked from our vehicles to a waiting area we saw two Ghanaian peacekeepers receiving first aid. They were brought over to our waiting area so they could be transported home for medical care. A brief glance at them told me they were in rough shape.

The Hercules landed a few minutes later. As usual, there was a mad dash to get everyone and everything on board. The frenetic activity was accompanied by a cacophony of sounds and smells—the cracking of gunfire mixed with the sound of plane engines, the smell of fuel. That day a tense- and concerned-looking General Dallaire was there to see everyone off. A nurse was on the flight, as per standard operating procedure, in case there were injured soldiers on board.

When the plane arrived a military policeman and a loadmaster stepped off. I rounded up my crew and allowed the two injured Ghanaians to be boarded first. As I made my way onto the plane the nurse was clipping the stretchers into their harnesses. In a case of bureaucratic foolishness, the military policeman stopped me, declaring that he couldn't take us on board if there were casualties on the flight. He was just doing his job, but rigidly applying peacetime rules in the middle of a war wasn't the most brilliant idea. Sometimes in the military common sense just doesn't prevail.

General Dallaire relied on these daily flights as an air bridge between Kenya and Rwanda, one that was especially crucial for bringing food and fresh water, which were always in short supply.* He looked visibly annoyed that a drawn-out conversation was now taking place: speed was clearly of the utmost importance. He approached the ramp and gave the poor corporal a dressing-down, telling him in no uncertain terms to get everyone on the plane and get the hell out of there. Looking embarrassed and cowed, the soldier stepped back and helped finish the loading process. The plane soon took off.

On board, the passengers were positioned on the right side of the plane, facing its centre, where the two Ghanaians were being cared for by a young female nurse, Leslie Newell. She was working frantically to save their lives. One of the men seemed fairly stable, but the other was severely injured, and the entire left side of his abdomen was exposed. For over an hour Leslie worked tirelessly while we sat and watched, helpless to do anything. Suddenly she just stopped. Resting her hands on the side of the stretcher, she looked at the floor and buried her head between her arms. The injured soldier, Private Mensah-Baidoo, who'd been hit when RPF shells landed on the Amahoro Stadium, had succumbed to his injuries.

That first week and a half in Rwanda had been full of high-intensity moments, but it was a surreal feeling to be on that flight, in a moment of relative calm, and witness firsthand the true impact of war. Look-

---

* Refugees and UN personnel alike sometimes went entirely without food and water for several days.

ing back on that moment, I can see that witnessing that man die was one of the first times that I really *experienced* the collateral damage of trauma—the injury to the brain; the subsequent mental erosion; the fatigue; the moral conflict. At the time none of that really sank in, but when I think about Leslie burying her head in her hands, I know that that experience was transformative. Like most people, I had dealt with adversity in my life, but this was a new type of stress, far beyond what people normally go through in the course of their lives.

For years afterward, whenever my thoughts drifted to Rwanda and the Ghanaian soldier's death, I wondered what became of Leslie. As luck would have it I ended up bumping into her down the road, when I worked on non-clinical mental health services for the Department of National Defence in 2008. We were by then both lieutenant-colonels. Leslie had always been a radiant individual with a good heart and kind eyes. But like many who served in Rwanda, the proximity to death had taken its toll. I could see through the stoic veneer that Canadian Forces members display in public that military service had eroded her spirit, just as it had mine. Not all of my colleagues were supportive of my work, but it was evident that Leslie was enthusiastic and extremely supportive of what I was doing (more on that later). After a great deal of pondering why that was the case, I inferred that she was so supportive because she probably knew *exactly* what it felt like to have a stress injury.

Chapter 2

THE RAVAGES OF WAR

After the Rwandan Civil War ended in July 1994 the humanitarian crisis was enormous. By the end of August over 2 million Rwandans were living in thirty-five different refugee camps scattered across various neighbouring countries, with an additional 300,000 in displaced persons camps within the country. Cholera, dysentery, and starvation were rampant in these crowded, squalid conditions. The camps were also dangerous because many of the Interahamwe and RGF soldiers used them to melt back into the civilian population, thereby escaping retribution at the hands of the victorious RPF. Some even used the camps as staging areas for future attempts to take back the country. On top of worrying about the population's health and safety, the UN and the new Rwandan government were also concerned with restarting the economy, especially the agricultural sector, which was the country's main source of food and exports.

As a way to get people out of the camps and back to some semblance of normal life, General Dallaire asked me to devise a way to communicate to the almost one million refugees in Goma, Zaire (now the Democratic Republic of Congo), on Rwanda's northwestern border, that it was safe to return. Goma lies just south of Mount Nyiragongo, an active volcano, which means the ground there is slow to absorb any moisture.* Since there were also very few sanitary facilities for the refugees to use, many in the five massive camps that had sprung up resorted to relieving themselves on the ground. The presence of urine and fecal matter contributed to all sorts of medical problems.

The age of the cell phone was still several years away in 1994, so most of the refugees initially had no idea the war was over. The challenge of convincing almost a million scared people to return home was compounded by the fact that many of them were illiterate, and so could not avail themselves of certain methods of communication. Initially I came up with the idea of airdropping single-frequency radios over the camps, through which the UN could broadcast messages, but the logistics were just too daunting. After consulting with various people and agencies who understood Rwandan culture better than I did, I devised a plan to produce several hundred thousand pamphlets. But that idea also presented challenges: in addition to high illiteracy rates, several different languages are spoken in Rwanda. I wasn't sure which one (or ones) the pamphlets should be in.

With the war over, flying in and out of the country was much easier, so I flew into Nairobi, where I found a talented Kenyan graphic artist well versed in East African culture. Together we brainstormed how to visually communicate the message I wanted to send. The final product had key words on one side in French and Kinyarwanda, another of Rwanda's official languages, for those who could read, and the other side contained straightforward images for those who couldn't. The basic message was this: it's safe to go home; if you stay here (in the camps) you will die; if you go home life can eventually return to some sort of normal rhythm. That was a tough message to have to send to

---

*   Nyiragongo eventually erupted in January 2002, killing 147 people and leaving 120,000 Congolese homeless. It is nonetheless fortuitous an eruption did not occur during the refugee crisis, or the casualty figures might have been even higher.

people who'd just witnessed death and destruction on a catastrophic scale, but it was necessary to save lives.

I was told the pamphlet's printing and production would take a little while, which was frustrating but understandable given the quantity involved. I returned to Rwanda to continue other work. Back in Kigali, I bumped into General Dallaire in a hallway of the Amahoro. Right away he asked me, "Have you airdropped those pamphlets yet?" I looked at him in despair. The printing industry in Rwanda, along with many of the people who worked in it, was dead, and going outside of the country meant there was no way to get the pamphlets made in less than a week; so far only three or four days had elapsed. But he was a general, and I understood the urgency of the situation, so I felt a mixture of worry and incompetence at my inability to answer him in the affirmative. Nonetheless, I explained that the pamphlets were in production, and that they would be dropped very soon. He understood, and we both had a bit of a laugh. I realized later that his question was a subtle way of putting pressure on one of his captains to speed things along.

A few days later the pamphlets arrived in several dozen boxes. To drop them, we decided to use a company called Canadian Helicopters, which had aircraft at Kigali Airport. The pilots, however, had a few concerns. The first was that the helicopter's slipstream would cause the pamphlets to be sucked back into the tail rotor, potentially causing an accident. After conducting several test runs we discovered that, as long as the helicopter maintained a certain altitude and speed, a person leaning out onto the aircraft's skid could thrust each "brick" of pamphlets downward, keeping them from being pulled into the slipstream.

At any rate, it was quite a sight to see hundreds of thousands of sheets of paper flying through the air like a thick cloud. I encountered some trouble, though, when I forgot to take the tie-wrap off one of the stacks of pamphlets. As if in slow motion, I can recall seeing an elderly man standing on the ground, waiting to catch the brick of paper as it fell from the sky. It came crashing down and hit him in the head a few seconds later. I saw him fall down, but given the helicopter's speed I

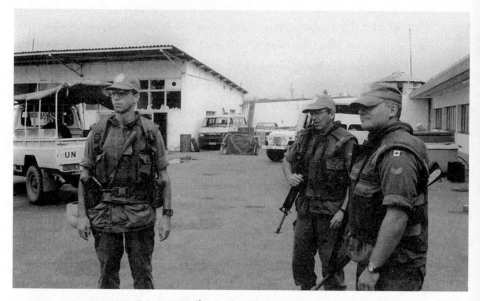

LEFT TO RIGHT: me, Warrant Officer John Blouin, and Corporal Chris Cassavoy, on the day of the pamphlet drop over Goma, Zaire (now Democratic Republic of Congo).

couldn't tell whether or not he'd been seriously injured, and I quickly lost sight of him in the hordes of people below. To this day I still hope that he wasn't seriously hurt by my mistake.

We were lucky that day, as neither the Interahamwe nor the RGF shot at us (or if they did, we couldn't tell with the noise of the helicopter's rotors). Once the last pamphlets were thrown we headed back to Kigali, where we landed less than an hour later. Unfortunately, we learned afterwards that, in spite of our preparation and hard work, the mission was a total failure. When they saw a UN helicopter with paper falling out of it, many of the refugees assumed we were throwing money. I'm not sure why they thought we would do that, since money was virtually useless in the country's war-ravaged economy (and throwing it out of a helicopter wouldn't exactly be an efficient way of dispensing it). But that is what they expected. And when they discovered that we were simply dropping pamphlets they were rather disappointed and upset with the UN. We also learned that members of the Interahamwe and the RGF sprinkled throughout the camp intimi-

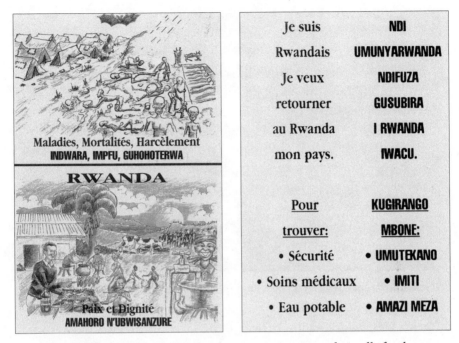

The pamphlet, front and reverse, with its message portrayed visually for those who could not read, as well as in both French and Kinyarwanda.

dated the small number of those already thinking about leaving. Such was the nature of operating in the fog of war, not to mention in places where cultural differences and our limited UN mandate caused so many unexpected headaches.

IN EARLY SEPTEMBER 1994, several weeks after the war and genocide had ended, there was a slew of activity as UN soldiers were deployed and humanitarian aid ramped up. With all of the changes taking place as the country transitioned to peace, we quickly realized that it was crucial to ensure that the sites of recent massacres be protected, photographed, studied, and documented, mainly to prevent any evidence from the genocide being lost. As human rights tribunals started gearing up, forensic investigators were starting to arrive in Rwanda to begin the overwhelming task of identifying the approximately 800,000 victims. The UN was not usually in the business of investigating

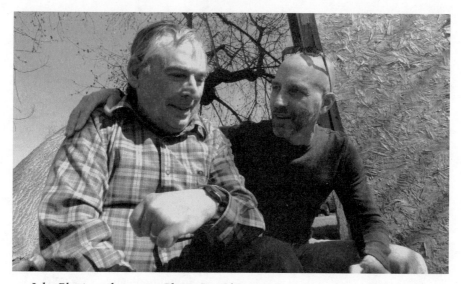

John Blouin and me, 2017. Photo: Jon O'Connor

genocides, but we wanted to help fill gaps wherever they existed. And, as with most of the peacekeeping operations the organization undertook in the 1990s, members of various UN contingents were eager to assist beyond the scope of our primary mandate. Since I had a photographer, John Blouin, working for me, and was now familiar with the country, I was called upon to help.

I soon joined a team that was tasked with finding a place called Ntarama, about an hour's drive northwest of Kigali, where a massacre took place on April 15, 1994. In Rwanda's urban areas, roads are paved and well looked after, but once we entered the countryside we were forced to travel small, single-lane dirt roads, often with trees on both sides. Adding to the difficulty, smaller towns and villages were not well marked on maps and they lacked the proper signage. That morning we set off for what was supposed to be an hour-long drive; instead we made it to Ntarama after three circuitous hours.

On the journey I was once again reminded of the recent genocide. I remember the beautiful, lush green countryside dotted with coffee and banana plantations—scenery whose breathtaking beauty belied the violence that had recently taken place. At one point during our drive we stopped for a short break. I used the opportunity to find a spot to relieve myself in the bush-line off the road. As I was looking for a spot my nostrils were suddenly filled with the stench of rotting flesh. I looked down and saw a severed human leg with pants and a boot still on it. Standing there, overwhelmed by the smell and the surreal nature of the scene before me, I thought to myself, "I guess we must be getting close to Ntarama." That smell has stayed with me ever since. Over the years morbidly inquisitive people have sometimes asked me to describe what rotting bodies smell like, and the best answer I can provide is that they smell oddly "spicy," for lack of a better word.

We got back in our vehicles and completed our journey to Ntarama, eventually arriving in an open field surrounded by trees. The local church, a red brick building, overlooked the village. We parked our vehicles in the knee-high grass, glanced around, and started walking toward the church. As we made our approach the grass gradually became flatter and flatter, and once we got a little closer to the church we understood why. The ground was completely littered with corpses, which from afar—because of months of rain, decomposition, and the tattered clothes the victims had been wearing—looked like dirt and garbage. Some bodies were grouped together while others lay on their own, perhaps because they tried to run away and were gunned down in the process. There were adults and children of all ages, several thousand of them.

Even among so many corpses, one that we found particularly shocking was the rotting body of a woman in an ankle-length skirt. She lay on her back, with her skirt lifted over her body and her legs spread apart. It immediately dawned on us that this woman, along with many others in the village, had been savagely raped before being killed. We continued on through the pungent smell of decaying bodies, many of which were in pieces. At one spot a head lay three feet from a body, and in another an arm lay several feet from a torso. As I surveyed the scene I found myself wondering which head fit with which body, and I guessed at the age of the children, who ranged from infants to teenagers. We weren't forensic experts and so couldn't touch anything—our job was simply to document what we found, do a basic count, and take some pictures so that the forensic teams had

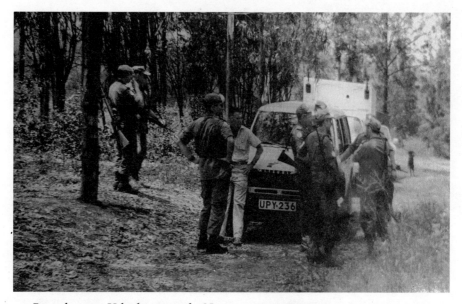

Rwanda, 1994: Vehicle stop at the Ntarama massacre site.

some recent evidence when they arrived. John Blouin started filming the scene and taking photos from different angles while I helped others do a body count and document what we saw.

After working in the field for a little while we approached the church. From the outside we noticed that there were a couple of large blast holes in the walls. When we looked through them into the church we saw what can only be described as hell on earth. Bodies were piled from wall to wall. Pews had been tipped over and scattered about the floor, and it was evident, even after just one glance, that people had tried all manner of jumping, moving, and dodging to escape their fate. They had sought refuge in the church because they believed that a holy place would provide protection, and because religious sites had traditionally been spared. But of course the Interahamwe didn't operate by any sort of conventional rules or principles. And in fact, we later found out from survivors that people had been told they should go to the church; the Interahamwe had allegedly planted this information to lure and concentrate people in one spot. Once the people were assembled, members of the militiamen locked the doors and shot rocket-propelled grenades at the church walls, to create open-

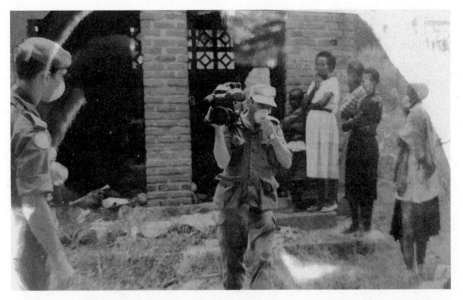

Warrant Officer John Blouin with his camera. Blouin documented hours and hours of evidence of the Rwandan genocide for human rights investigators.

ings through which to shoot people and throw hand grenades. Given what we saw, this story made sense.

We documented the scene inside the church through these blast holes. It was eerily quiet as we went about our grim business, and none of us spoke. This wasn't necessarily out of respect for the people who'd been killed, although I'm sure that was part of it. For my part, I was quiet because the scene was just so completely and utterly surreal. I had arrived at a place, both physically and mentally, where I now realized the full extent of what humans can do to each other because of ethnicity or other perceived differences. Coming from Quebec, where talk of the ethnic differences between French and English Canadians were particularly heated in the 1990s, I thought at that moment about how bad things can get when humans lose track of the fact that, at the end of the day, we're all just flesh and blood. To have such disregard for life; to perpetrate an act like this—this was beyond any comprehension.

The sheer number of bodies inside the church made it virtually impossible to walk in without disturbing the site, so we documented what we could from the outside and turned over our evidence to the forensic experts. They would have the even more gruesome task of going through the pockets and belongings of thousands of decomposing corpses to try and identify the victims and provide a total body count.

I subsequently ended up back at Ntarama several times over the following months; since I was part of the team that had originally found the massacre site, I was able to guide delegates and forensic teams back there. Each time I returned the victims' bodies had reached a new stage of decomposition: it was as if time itself wanted to forget about what had happened there. The site is now a genocide museum and memorial centre, one of six such institutions in the country. Long after my tour I saw a picture of the Ntarama memorial on the Internet, one that depicted an ensemble of skulls. While looking at it I couldn't help but think: "Wow, I was one of the first people in the world to witness that." One doesn't easily forget such evil.

THE HUMANITARIAN CRISIS worsened after the war ended in July 1994 due to the damage done to the country's economy and infrastructure. Much of the population was dead, food was in short supply, medical care was almost nonexistent, and people were dispersed all over the country and beyond. Various UN contingents were deployed around Rwanda to try and ameliorate the situation. Canada had two major teams handling different tasks throughout the remainder of 1994. The First Canadian Signal Regiment, a team of communication experts, was given the task of setting up communication relay stations in the mountains to ensure that various UN contingents scattered across the country could talk with one another. The second contingent was made up of a field ambulance unit deployed near Rwanda's western border to help provide medical care. Villages were empty, and many larger settlements looked like ghost towns. Although the violence had largely stopped, things were still unstable as the country tried to recover some kind of equilibrium.

In the late summer I was part of a convoy sent to visit and lend any assistance we could to an ad hoc orphanage that had no electricity, no running water, and limited food. We arrived after a long drive from Kigali at a compound resembling a monastery, with a series of similar-looking small buildings. When we got close it was obvious that the orphanage's inhabitants were in a bad state. There were about half a dozen adults there caring for hundreds of children who were sick, dehydrated, and in some cases on the verge of death. We had two medics with us, and they promptly started helping as best they could. I noticed a little boy who looked about seven or eight years old sitting on a cement step. He was naked except for a very large T-shirt that partially covered his bottom half. His elbows were resting on his knees and he just glanced around, seeming dazed and confused. Upon closer inspection I could see that his hands were totally maimed. His fingers, which were still attached but mangled and misshapen, were sticking out in all different directions. Like his country, he had been through hell.

I spoke with a woman who seemed like she was one of the people in charge; I asked her what had happened to the boy. She told me that when the Interahamwe showed up they tortured him with machetes. Without proper medical care or surgical knowledge, the best the women at the orphanage could come up with was to put his hands into a fire to cauterize the wounds. I cannot imagine what kind of pain that must have caused him. The women's action saved the boy's life, but his hands were severely burnt, and his fingers were fused in different positions. Without the use of his hands he would have a very difficult struggle in a place where most jobs involved physical labour and where there was no social safety net. Halfway through our conversation the woman suggested that, since I was Canadian, perhaps I could operate on him. I told her that I was not a doctor, and that his hands would require major surgery that even Canadian doctors could not perform in Rwanda.

But I wondered if there was some way I could help the boy. My father had recently retired, so when I called home a week later I told him of the boy's condition and asked if he could make some inquiries with some doctors in his area about what might be done to help. He agreed and started doing some research the next day. Eventually, he connected with the Shriners Hospital for Children in Montreal. I sent him pictures of the boy, which he brought to doctors there. They said that his hands would perhaps require multiple surgeries, but that it was certainly something they could do. After hearing the good news, my father and I started the long and labyrinthine process of trying to get the child to Canada—a project that took almost the entire remainder of my Rwanda deployment, from September 1994 to March 1995.

When I first met the boy in the late summer of 1994 there weren't many NGOs in Rwanda, so he was put in an orphanage while I exchanged paperwork with the Canadian and Rwandan immigration services. I was eventually visited in the fall of 1994 at the Amahoro by two women who worked for an Irish NGO that was aiding Rwandan children. They tried to convince me that sending the child to Canada was a bad idea. Their rationale was that Rwanda was his home, and that taking him away from his culture would be detrimental to his upbringing. That meeting tipped me off to how the UN culture, which by the end of my tour included over three hundred NGOs working in Rwanda, sometimes operated.

Though I'm sure that they, too, wanted to help the child, I also had the impression that part of the women's rationale for keeping him in Rwanda was to have him as a poster boy to help with their fundraising activities. Why else would an NGO be so concerned with one particular child, especially when there were thousands of others also needing their help?

The answer, I believed, was simple. Rwanda was an even less hot topic than it had been during the genocide a few months earlier, so many agencies leveraged certain individual cases so as to maximize their fundraising capabilities. I guess that's how they felt they had to operate, but I still found it very distasteful. Given the progress I had made in getting the boy some help, and the somewhat illusory ability of those women to ensure he received the surgery he needed, I told them I was pressing on. I thanked them, and left the meeting with the impression that they weren't happy with my decision.

In the meantime, my father had been trying to find a family in Canada to sponsor the child. After calling various agencies and individuals he found a potential candidate in Lachute. Given that this was my birthplace, it felt like fate—after all, what were the odds? The family, the Carrières, had adopted many children in the past, and they were in many ways the archetypal Good Samaritans. Without any coaxing they agreed to sponsor the boy, further increasing his chances of a better life.

In the late fall of 1994 I visited the boy again, and this time I brought a medic with me; the fear of HIV/AIDS was palpable throughout the Western world in the 1990s, and I had to ensure he was tested for the virus before he came to Canada. Fortunately the test came back negative. I breathed a sigh of relief, carried on with my daily work, and waited for word on the boy's application.

Despite my best efforts, though, the boy was still in Rwanda when my tour ended in March 1995. The Shriners Hospital was ready to operate and the Carrière family was ready to accept him, but both the Rwandan and Canadian governments had dragged their heels, as governments often do. I had put so much work into seeing the boy get the surgery he needed, and I wanted to see things through to the end. But helping him was a personal mission, not part of my job as a UN peacekeeper. There was nothing I could do now that my tour was up. So I left Rwanda with a very heavy heart, feeling for all intents and purposes like I'd failed.

Two years later, in the spring of 1997 I was at work at NDHQ in Ottawa when my father called to inform me of some good news. After I left Rwanda a Canadian priest who'd found the child heard about my attempts to get him out of the country. He helped tie up some of the loose ends I was unable to rectify and managed to get the boy to Canada. My father, who'd likewise lost track of the child's status, heard the news through my mother's extended family, who he still visited from time to time. The boy was now in Lachute with the Carrière family, and his surgeries were only a few weeks away. Since my father was coming to visit me that weekend, he suggested that we visit the family and thank them.

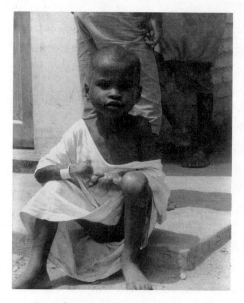

Rwanda, 1994: Ziragobora, when I first met him at the orphanage.

Meeting the Carrières and their new adopted son was like a dream. The boy, who'd grown a few inches since I'd last seen him, didn't remember me, but that didn't take away from the joy of knowing he was safe. During our visit, we had a few laughs over his penchant for flicking light switches off and on, even while people were in the room. He enjoyed it, I'm sure, both because it was an activity he could do with his injured hands, and also because indoor electricity was new to him. The Carrières asked me if I wanted to continue my involvement with the boy's case, but I saw that he was in good hands and politely declined. I was happy just to see that the mission to get him to Canada had finally been accomplished.

Jumping ahead to 2011, I heard through the media that the boy—now a young man—was still living in Quebec, and that he'd authored a book about his life experiences, *Le Journal de Ziragobora*. I looked him up on the Internet and found a video of an interview he gave to a Quebec radio station. To my shock and surprise, he operated a Blackberry with his thumbs during the interview. It was a simple but heart-warming sign that the boy from Rwanda, whom during my tour I knew only as Ziragobora, his Kinyarwandan name, was alive and had found a better life in Canada. His name is now Jean Carrière and he lives in Quebec to this day.

DURING THE CIVIL war numerous Rwandan civilians and foreign expats sought refuge at the Centre Christus, an old Jesuit monastery (now a "spirituality centre") in the Kigali suburbs. The beautiful, well-groomed grounds evoked feelings of peace and serenity. But when the genocide began in April 1994 the centre was the scene of some of the first killings.

In early September 1994 I was brought by a local man to a small home on the centre's grounds. He explained to me what had happened in April before showing me the inside of a bedroom. There was dried blood all over the walls and floor, and the place was littered with empty AK-47 cartridges. It looked to me like the house's inhabitants had been killed while sleeping or relaxing.

A few weeks later I was looking for a German freelance journalist who'd asked me to obtain clearance for him to speak with RGF officials. Since many journalists and expats could often be found at the centre, I went to look for him there. When I arrived I decided to check the main hall first, since I had visited enough times to be recognized and might find help from one of the employees. As I parked my jeep I saw a man whom I recognized and had said hello to a few times; he was running towards me in a panicked state. His arms were in the air and he kept loudly repeating, "It's terrible! It's terrible!" He said that he needed the UN and he insisted that I follow him. Taken aback, I went with him to the edge of the parking lot, trying to calm him down as we walked. I thought perhaps he had found a corpse and wanted to show me. Sadly, corpses were nothing new to me by this point.

We went past the main hall to a trail that snaked around the centre grounds. The trail was comprised of two dirt tire tracks separated by a grassy hump; he walked down the left side and I walked beside him on the right. After about fifty metres he stopped, pointed to the ground, and yelled, "Look! Look! Look! This is where it exploded!" Just beside the trail at the base of a tree was a crater about four feet wide and two feet deep. When I asked him what, exactly, had exploded, he replied, "Children!"

It turned out that two kids had been playing in the area when one of them accidentally stepped on a land mine. He died instantly, and his friend lost an eye. By the time I'd arrived several hours had passed since the incident, but when I examined the crater I could still see coagulated blood amid the rust-coloured soil. At that moment I looked up at the man and my blood boiled, not from sadness or pity but from anger. All I could think was, "There are mines here. He brought us into a fucking minefield." As soon as the realization hit me I yelled for him to stay where he was. Of course, when I explained that we were likely standing in a minefield he became extremely nervous.

By the time the war in Afghanistan started in 2001, Canadian military personnel were receiving training on how to get out of minefields, but in the mid-1990s we knew nothing about this. Rightly or wrongly, I decided that since we'd come up the trail without harm it was probably the safest way to return. I told the man to get onto the trail in as few steps as possible, and we commenced our walk back toward the centre. As had happened on many occasions during my time in Rwanda, I felt an electric current shoot up and down my spine as I slowly walked back, not knowing if one wrong step was going to kill or seriously injure me. Thankfully, we arrived back at the parking lot, and I told the man not to venture off the centre's grounds again. That felt like one of the longest walks of my life.

Afterwards I drove back to the Amahoro complex and spoke with Captain Jerry Deveaux, the man in charge of the Canadian Forces engineers. The engineers, a great bunch of guys, had their work cut out for them: it was their job to remove all of the mines, unexploded mortar rounds, and other cheap explosive ordnance scattered around Kigali during the war. Deveaux was a seasoned veteran and a calm leader. He listened patiently to my story. When I was finished, he said matter-of-factly that I should take him to the spot. I brought him to the centre and showed him the parallel grooves I'd walked with the Rwandan man. We took the same path to the mine crater.

About halfway there Jerry told me to stop. I immediately halted and looked at him. He crouched down, staring at the ground in front of him, then calmly told me to back up. I took several reverse steps. Lightly, he rubbed the ground just in front of where my right foot had been. A flat piece of metal appeared; "TS-50" was engraved on it. Jerry took out his knife, scraped away the packed dirt, and popped out a sand-coloured TS-50 anti-personnel mine. He stood up again, looked at me, and said that it was my lucky day. Somehow the Rwandan man and I had been on that path twice and narrowly missed stepping on it. If Jerry hadn't removed the mine, more innocent people could've been maimed or killed.

Jerry laughed off my close call, and at the time I did, too. Looking back, though, I realize how close I came to disaster. The engineers went to the centre a few days later and found about a dozen mines scattered around the area. They told me that it was common for the warring armies to place land mines at the base of trees, since trees provided shelter from the heat of the sun and were a natural resting spot for tired soldiers. Many people—soldiers and civilians alike—must have gone to sit down beside a tree for a rest, not knowing that it was going to be the last moment of their life.

AROUND THIS TIME, in the early fall of 1994, I was assigned a driver, Corporal Chris Cassavoy. Along with John Blouin, I was in touch with Chris regularly throughout the fall. We all lived and worked out of the Amahoro, and at the end of each day it was common for us to shoot the breeze about the week's events.

One afternoon I was thinking that I hadn't seen Chris in a day or two when, less than an hour later, he showed up; he was visibly disturbed and shaken up. John and I asked him how he was doing, but it was difficult to gauge how he was feeling at first. He was always joking around, and sure enough, though he looked upset he was still cracking jokes. In 1994 the Canadian military was oblivious to post-traumatic stress disorder and what we now call stress injuries. Like other junior officers, I had received no sensitivity training or briefings about mental health—in short, I was part of the problem. Nonetheless, after a few moments Chris walked into our sleeping quarters and put his head in his hands, saying he had just had the worst experience of his life. After collecting his thoughts he began to relate what had happened.

Early that afternoon Chris was driving back to the Amahoro on a Kigali side road when he came upon a three-way junction that connected with the main road to the airport and stadium. Approaching from the right, he joined a group of vehicles that, unbeknownst to him—they were of various makes and models and weren't clearly marked—was actually a Rwandan government convoy.

All of a sudden the vehicles in front of him came to a screeching halt while simultaneously the ones behind accelerated, sandwiching Chris in between. A tall, angry-looking Rwandan army officer quickly jumped out of one of the vehicles in front and walked towards Chris's jeep. Unsure of what was going on, Chris began to exit his vehicle, but as he was getting out the officer pushed the door back on him, wedging him in. In French the officer castigated Chris for coming between the convoy's vehicles. Chris, who was an anglophone with little knowledge of French, caught only some of the man's diatribe; he was still unsure of the exact problem.

As the officer poked Chris's chest, Chris noticed that he was now surrounded by soldiers pointing their AK-47s at him. He stood there helplessly for a few minutes as the officer yelled at him. Knowing that if he reached for his own rifle he might be killed, Chris took the man's abuse and hoped for the best. Then, just as suddenly as they'd appeared, the men got back into their vehicles and drove off, leaving Chris shocked and overwhelmed.

While relating the story Chris's face grew quite red: he was clearly disturbed by what he'd experienced. John and I listened, but we were at a loss for things to say. We weren't trained in how to handle those types of events, nor did I really understand the effects of any of this on myself or others. By that point I'd seen countless horrific things and had several brushes with death—I assumed Chris's experience amounted to just another bad day at the office. All John and I knew how to do was make jokes about it and carry on with our work.

This might sound like a cliché, but I really wish I had known then what I know now. I don't necessarily think I would have done anything different that day, but I would have at least known to follow up with Chris, to ask him how he was doing. I should've pulled him aside a couple days later and asked how he was handling things; that would have given him the opportunity to talk about his experience if he wanted to. Even if he struggled with things down the road I could have connected with him and let him know he didn't have to face the harrowing event in his own head, alone.

Instead, I was completely oblivious. I still hadn't been equipped with the ability to recognize when a colleague was having a hard time and to engage with them in a person-to-person manner. After Rwanda, Chris's experience, and my (mis)handling of it, weighed on me. The incident demonstrated the importance of being able to connect with someone when they're dealing with hardships. It shaped my thoughts and future work in numerous ways.

Another experience from this period showed me just how much the cumulative stress of dealing with horrific events can affect people over time. In November 1994 Chris and John travelled with several Canadian intelligence officers to a school in the southeastern part of Rwanda that during the genocide had been the site of a massacre. Once again they were tasked with exploring and documenting what they saw.

Initially they couldn't spot any signs of what had taken place in the school, but the evidence wasn't far away. When Chris walked into the long grass on the edge of the site he noticed something underfoot. He looked down and discovered that his boot had sunken into the chest cavity of a corpse. Frightened and disturbed, he attempted to leap away, but as he did so he tripped and rolled into a hole containing a pile of bodies. Along with being held and threatened by the Rwandan government convoy, it was another experience that, in retrospect, probably affected Chris long afterward, even though at the time it was seen as just another hard day at work. I could see Chris, and myself, gradually looking more tired, haggard, and vacant from being involved in many similar events like this, but we didn't know enough to connect these experiences to our deteriorating mental states.

AROUND THIS TIME there was a short lull in my own work, so I decided to take advantage of the respite and go on the hike of a lifetime. The Virunga Mountains, a series of volcanoes along Rwanda's northern border, are home to some of the most breathtaking scenery in the world. But even more intriguing than the mountains themselves was the possibility of spotting the elusive and endangered mountain gorillas made famous by murdered American zoologist Dian Fossey, whose story captivated me after I watched the 1988 movie *Gorillas in the Mist*.

I left the Amahoro early one morning with John Blouin and a few other Canadian comrades, and we were headed to the Rwanda-Zaire border. After a few hours we veered off the main (paved) road and arrived at a small village close to the base of the mountains. It was a very rural place, with tiny homes made of packed mud and covered with straw roofs. I couldn't be certain, but it appeared from its tranquil look and lack of any obvious destruction that the village may have been spared the horrors that had recently devastated most of the country.

We didn't really know where we were going, and the tourism industry was still in shambles, so we had to find a local guide to direct us. With the local economy being what it was, it didn't take us long to find a guide and negotiate a reasonable price. At first it was difficult to tell whether he was being truthful about being a guide before the war, but he seemed like our best chance, so we gave him a shot. Thankfully, he was not only truthful but a kind and gentle soul. Since we were both francophones, I had the privilege of speaking with him during our ascent.

We began the long climb up around lunchtime, and although everyone was in good shape, the going was tough, largely due to the slippery, muddy terrain, which sometimes made it difficult to maintain our footing. The trail was very narrow—just wide enough for one person—and in some areas we had to walk with one foot directly in front of the other.

The first thing that amazed me as we ascended was the vegetation, a lush deep green. The jungle's sheer fecundity was somewhat dreamlike, and it immediately took me back to the old Tarzan movies of my childhood. There was only one lookout along the trail from which to gaze off into the distance; the thick canopy of trees and other vegetation covered us entirely the rest of the way. As we climbed higher and higher the flora began to change, and we started seeing gorilla feces. There were thousands of green plants everywhere, all with long stems protruding out of the ground. They had the feel of a stalk of celery and they snapped very easily, making it almost impossible to walk quietly, as per our guide's instructions. With the noise we were making I was almost certain we had scared off every gorilla within a ten-kilometre radius, but I kept my fingers crossed. Eventually, we found a small clearing and sat down in silence, hoping the gorillas would pass through the area in spite of our clumsiness.

To our surprise, after about ten minutes several gorillas emerged from the jungle. Amazingly, though some were quite immense, they ambled silently through the same vegetation we had just crashed through like bulls in a China shop. They ranged in size from babies all the way up to one massive silverback. After a few minutes they came within twenty feet of us and began eating the vegetation; except for the silverback, who kept his distance, they eyed us with what looked like a mix of curiosity and caution.

What happened next will always stay with me. One juvenile gorilla, glancing mischievously at us, seemed to want to show off his tree-climbing skills. He kept running and swinging off a tree branch and returning to his mother. After several repetitions he grabbed hold of a branch and began hanging upside down, seemingly taunting us with his strength and agility. But suddenly he lost his grip and fell down onto the vegetation below. When he got up he was uninjured, but it was evident that his pride had taken a hit. He demonstrated an incredibly human-like demeanour as he looked at us again, then at the ground, in what looked like embarrassment; it was as if he wanted to know if we'd witnessed his fall. Chastened by the experience, he walked over to cuddle with his mother, as a young boy does after discovering the power of gravity. We laughed quietly and continued to watch the gorillas for about thirty minutes. Eventually they moved to another area. I could think only of the magic of what we'd witnessed as we continued on our trek.

The Virunga trip was capped by a visit to Dian Fossey's research laboratory, located between Mount Karisimbi and Mount Bisoke. Although Fossey had been murdered almost ten years earlier, in 1985,

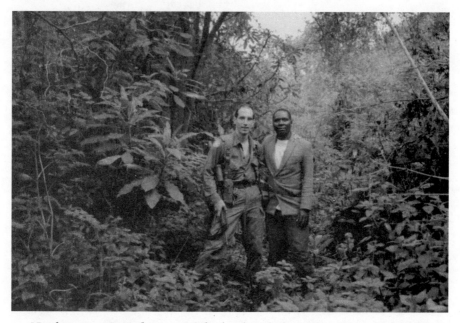

North-western Rwanda, 1994: With a local guide during my visit to the Mount Karisimbi region.

her lab was still largely intact. There was a padlock on the door, but visitors could look through the windows and see her research tools and living area, which were more or less frozen in time. I spotted a few microscopes, some glass jars and beakers, as well as some basic tools hanging on the wall. What struck me was just how austere the lab was, in sharp contrast to the archetypal science lab, with its white floors and polished stainless steel. It must have taken true dedication to live and work in these conditions, so far from any town or people. Outside of the lab, the crosses marking the graves Fossey made for slain gorillas were still there as well. I managed to get a picture of myself beside the grave of Digit, Fossey's favourite gorilla, whose death at the hands of poachers in 1978 inspired her to create the Digit Fund (now the Dian Fossey Gorilla Fund International) to raise money for anti-poaching patrols.

The entire outing was very dreamlike. The mountains were a world away from everything that had occurred in the country below. That trip was truly a once-in-a-lifetime opportunity, and probably the

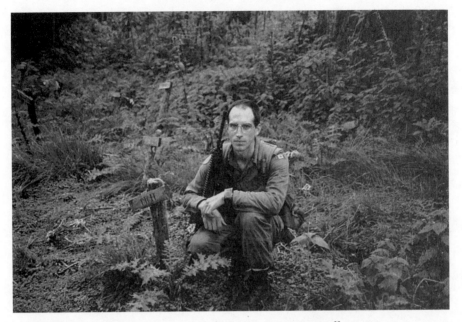

At the grave of Digit, Dian Fossey's favourite mountain gorilla.

best—perhaps the only—thing I did for my mental health during my ten months in Rwanda. Unfortunately, as we made the trek back to the base of the mountains reality hit me like a ton of bricks: I was still in Rwanda; I would have to endure several more months of tragedy.

A SHORT TIME after Chris's chest-cavity incident I was with John Blouin, at the same school where Chris had discovered the bodies, once again collecting evidence. The first sign we found of the recent genocide was the unmistakable smell of dead bodies.

On one side of the compound we saw several stairs leading up to a rectangular cement structure. At first glance it looked like the foundation of a building that had not yet been built. When we got closer we could see that, while it was only about ten feet wide, it was quite deep, like a well. With every step we took, the smell of death grew stronger; it reached a peak as we stood at the structure's edge and looked in. About fifteen feet down, at the bottom of the hole, was a pool of water, and sitting within it was a pile of bodies.

After staring into the hole for a few moments we continued looking for more spots that needed documenting. When we were certain we'd finished combing the area, we investigated the small, single-story classroom buildings. In the first we found pieces of broken furniture and burnt objects strewn all over the floor. Then the real shock came: there were brown streaks of coagulated blood all over the walls, as if someone had waved a wet paint brush. On the ground we noticed several large, circular blood stains, evidently where the victims lay while they succumbed to their wounds. The Interahamwe had a habit of using machetes to kill people, and from what we gathered it appeared that they had hacked their victims numerous times before leaving them to die. The corpses that Chris Cassavoy had previously rolled onto, and the ones we saw inside the cement well, were more than likely the victims whose blood we now stared at.

Chapter 3

THE TIPPING POINT

As the tour dragged on I noticed that I was starting to lose my grip.

The war had been over for several months in November 1994, and Kigali Airport was no longer the free-for-all it had been during the conflict. During the war, I simply drove my jeep right up to a plane or helicopter whenever I needed to catch a flight, but now it was necessary to go through various security measures. The helicopter hangars used by the UN were on the far side of the airport's single landing strip. We could access them by either circumventing the entire airport and taking a long dirt road through various townships—a journey that took almost an hour—or we could take the much easier route we'd become accustomed to over the last several months: driving across the runway.

Several weeks had elapsed since I had last taken a chopper, so I wasn't aware that new security measures had been put in place. On the day in question I was to go with the Canadian UN commander who'd replaced General Dallaire, Major-General Guy Tousignant, to visit the UN's Ethiopian battalion. They had just killed several former RGF members, who they'd caught stealing cows—an excessive use of force for the theft of livestock that certainly wouldn't help the UN's cause. Given his position and stature, General Tousignant had his own convoy and could come and go from the airport as he pleased. I, on the other hand, was a captain; I needed to go through various protocols to board a flight.

General Tousignant and I had arranged to meet at the airport, so I started driving there about an hour before our flight departed. When I arrived I was surprised to find myself in front of armed soldiers and barricades. There was nothing inherently alarming about this, of course, since it signalled the country's slow stabilization, but for my purposes it meant I could no longer take the shortcut across the runway. In the distance I could see that General Tousignant's convoy had already reached the helicopter hangars: I would now be the last to arrive. I tried to negotiate my way through the security gate outside, but the guards insisted I go inside the terminal and obtain special permission to cross the runway. I didn't want to make my commander wait (that is seriously frowned upon in the military), but I had no choice. The guards told me to park my car and head inside. I complied, and started walking toward the terminal.

When I got to the doors two armed guards with AK-47s stepped in front of me and told me that I couldn't go in. When I asked why they pointed to my pistol, which sat under my arm in its shoulder holster. I was a bit puzzled. I was a UN representative, and although under normal circumstances it might seem foolish to show up at an airport with a pistol on display, this had been common practice for UN soldiers throughout my time in Rwanda.

With the clock ticking I became exasperated. The younger of the two guards wouldn't give up, and told me I could only enter if I surrendered my weapon. As a soldier and UN representative I found his request disagreeable, and I told him I couldn't comply. The conversation quickly descended into a contest of wills. I pointed to the desk I needed to get to, and told him he could accompany me if he liked. He refused. I took my right hand and gently pushed him out of the way and said that I didn't have time for his obstruction. As I walked past he turned and yelled "STOP!" before cocking his weapon and pointing it at my chest. Firmly, he told me that if I didn't halt, he would shoot.

Under normal circumstances, which is to say before my time in Rwanda, I would never have played chicken with a large, heavily armed guard. But something strange had taken over my mind, and in my present state his threat meant nothing to me—I just didn't care. And so I kept walking. He repeated his threat, this time even louder. It was then that I experienced the return of the sensation I'd felt a few times before, something like an electric current surging up and down my spine. It was like a premonition, as if my body was expecting— perhaps wanted—a bullet to penetrate it.

At that late stage of my tour I was no longer acting sensibly. I felt no fear of death, and in some ways I think I even longed for it. I had lost any idea of how to calibrate risk, indeed whether to care about risk at all. I didn't understand or bother to weigh the dangers of what I was experiencing. I was now of the opinion that, if the war and what I'd witnessed hadn't killed me, what could this man possibly do? The entire situation somehow felt meaningless. All that mattered at that moment was the task I had to accomplish, and the man pointing his gun at me was simply in the way. There was no way I was going to miss my chopper ride, even if it meant ignoring a man with an AK-47.

In the end no shots were fired; the guard backed down, and I won our battle of wills. I obtained my piece of paper and walked out of the terminal. The young man was, of course, livid: I'd defied him and gotten away with it. When I left the terminal and climbed into my jeep, I wondered to myself for a few short minutes, "What just happened?" But I just shrugged and carried on as if nothing significant had happened. I gave my paper to the guards outside, crossed the runway, and parked my jeep with five minutes to spare. General Tousignant glanced at his watch as I approached, no doubt thinking that I'd made it just in the nick of time. We got into the helicopter and in a few minutes were on our way.

The recklessness I'd demonstrated with the young Rwandan guard was a testament to how impeded my judgement had become. My fine-tuned sense of risk had disappeared. The perverse effect of this

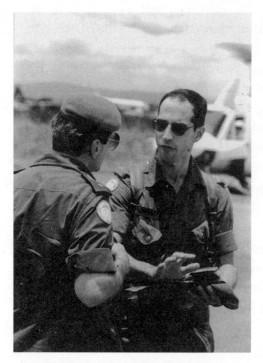

With Major-General Guy Tousignant during our field visit with the UN's Ethiopian battalion. Tousignant had replaced Romeo Dallaire as force commander in August 1994.

transformation was a high like nothing I'd ever felt. Taking undue risks now provided a drug-like surge. But like most drugs, the high didn't last long, and instead of providing me with lasting sustenance, it left me an adrenalin junkie. I now lived for the next moment when my heart was going to jump out of my chest; I wanted to feel that electric current running up my spine. With hindsight, I know it was the first sign that I'd reached my tipping point.

The second sign came in December 1994, when I was tasked with escorting UN civilian workers on a long drive to the Tanzanian border. The RPF had allegedly committed some retaliatory killings in the area, and the UN wanted to look into them.

It may have been overly cautious of me, but during the early days of my deployment I'd developed a driving habit that some of us called a "rolling halt." The rolling halt involved putting the jeep in neutral and turning it off as I approached potential danger. The jeep continued moving but without making a sound, which allowed me to hear if there was any gunfire or strange noises ahead. If there *was*, I could simply turn the car back on and drive away. Because hostilities had ceased by this point (open hostilities at least), there really was no reason for me to take precautions like this anymore. But like some of my other habits, the rolling halt was ingrained after months of navigating risky situations.

Our destination on the Tanzanian border was in a low, grassy area. When we arrived I was going about forty kilometres an hour. I put the car in neutral, turned the engine off, and let the jeep glide for several seconds. As the vehicle slowly came to a stop we began to hear loud cracking and popping sounds underneath the tires. A bit puzzled, we climbed out of the vehicle and looked to see where the noises were emanating from. One of the civilians looked down at the ground and turned to me with a mix of abhorrence and terror on her face. "Oh my God," she said. "We just rolled over some human remains. Bones— that's probably the sound we heard!"

I replied, somewhat dismissively: "That's nothing, you should hear the sound of rolling over a skull—it *really* pops." Everyone stopped and stared at me, then looked at one another, somewhat shocked by my flippant response. Things were understandably awkward for a few moments after that. But after the initial shock, along with my unnerving response, had worn off, everyone carried on with their tasks. We drove back to Kigali later that evening.

That night at the Amahoro I was brushing my teeth before bed when, suddenly, my mind went into a loop. For about ten minutes I brushed away while working my way through some unpleasant thoughts and emotions—namely, my intense guilt and shame over being so disrespectful when driving over human bones.

Was it bravado? Was I trying to make light of a disturbing situation? I don't know. But when the human psyche reaches a certain point, when atrocity and extreme degradation become commonplace, certain defence mechanisms are put into play. People often display a dark sense of humour in an attempt to draw some form of relief out of even the most terrible scenes.* This dark humour serves as a sort of shield or mask, helping one to deflect and cope with bad situations. My sardonic response on the Tanzanian border was my way

---

* This phenomenon is well documented, especially by military histories concerning major wars or peacekeeping operations. Interested readers can direct themselves to Samuel Hynes's *The Soldiers' Tale: Bearing Witness to Modern War.*

of leveraging that sense of humour to protect myself, to prevent my mind from dealing with the fact that I was on the very ground where approximately 800,000 people had recently been slaughtered.

At the time these realizations were still far off in the distance. That night, I just brushed my teeth while feeling extremely guilty about how I'd acted. Afterward I went to bed and lay silently on my cot, staring at the mosquito net around my bed. As I drifted off to sleep I asked myself, "What's wrong with me? Why the hell would I say something like that?" I didn't have an answer, but at least I knew enough to ask the question.

I would think about these questions more and more in the ensuing years. Over time, I came to see that day on the Tanzanian border as another piece of the puzzle that was my mental health. Wouldn't it be nice for future generations to have answers to the types of questions I'd asked myself that night at the Amahoro without needing years of distance and mental turmoil? I came to believe that we need to provide people with a new narrative, one that focuses on *behaviour* rather than *symptoms*. Dark humour is a manifestation of an underlying issue that *may* turn into a complex mental health problem down the road. If people knew where that tipping point—or points—lay, they could recognize sooner how to spot a change in themselves.

In the twenty-first century we hear a lot of talk about educating people and increasing their "mental health literacy." That is a great path to go on, but not necessarily when it involves using only clinical language. Instead, it's better to use tangible examples and replace clinical-sounding terms with regular, everyday analogies so that those with a basic understanding of mental health can spot early warning signs on their own.

IN JANUARY 1995, near the end of my tour, I was working at UNHQ for the UN secretary-general's special representative and General Tousignant. Over the past few months the UN had taken a strong public stance against possible retaliatory killings by the Tutsi-dominated RPF. We'd received numerous reports in the late summer and fall of 1994 that people from Hutu tribes had disappeared. Rumours were also cir-culating that hundreds of bodies were being burned and disposed of in Akagera National Park, in the northeastern part of the country. At one point General Tousignant, myself, and a military policeman took a helicopter flight over the park to determine if there was any evidence behind these claims. The park is huge, covering 1,200 square kilome-tres, so it was a bit like looking for a needle in a haystack, but we had to investigate nonetheless. The search was conducted largely to demon-strate that the UN was committed to preventing further genocide. In the end, we found no evidence to substantiate what we'd heard.

A few weeks earlier, in December 1994, I had recently been quoted by reporters while speaking on behalf of the UN, saying that we would not stand idly by if genocidal activities occurred again. This stance evidently riled the RPF liaison officers and government members, who'd won the civil war and were now keen to burnish their image as benevolent rulers, regardless of the fact that they, too, had been guilty of war crimes and the targeting of UN officials. One man in particular, a major whom we had gotten to know both during and after the war, was quite upset with my statement.

One day, after visiting General Tousignant at UNHQ, he stopped by my office for a chat. Sitting down at my desk, he opined that it was inappropriate for the UN to put pressure on the Rwandan government when there were only allegations—and no proof—that genocide was taking place. He also said that the UN had to change its stance, and that the Rwandan government would not tolerate any provoca-tion. He leaned forward as he spoke, clearly attempting to intimidate me. The major ended his monologue by telling me in no uncertain terms that Rwanda was a very "interesting" country, that people were known to die once in a while, and that even I, a UN representative, should not feel that I was immune to that particular fate. He stood up to leave, and told me with a stern look that I should watch my back. After he left my office I sat there for a few minutes, slightly stunned. I reported the conversation to my colleagues and General Tousignant. From what I gathered, I was the only one who'd been subjected to such thinly veiled threats.

The country was by this point relatively stable, with UN troops present in large numbers, so I had turned my pistol in to the quartermaster. But after being threatened by the RPF officer, I was told I should rearm myself just in case. That afternoon I drove to the field logistics unit several kilometres away to obtain another sidearm, but when I got there I was told by the major in charge that no more pistols were available; a new UN contingent had recently arrived and every available pistol was already issued. A master corporal listening to our conversation asked me why I needed a pistol, and after hearing my story, he offered to turn his in so one would become available. I thanked him, left with the pistol, and carried it with me for the rest of my tour. I wasn't exactly scared of the RPF officer's threats. I was, however, certainly anxious and paranoid. For the last several weeks of my deployment I looked behind me everywhere I went. When I drove anywhere I was likewise wary of any large vehicles or armed soldiers, and I was always wondering if people knew who I was or if they meant to do me harm.

Since I wasn't part of a larger unit I was usually alone, which further heightened my anxiety. My living situation also contributed to the stress. In late January I had been moved from the Amahoro to a place called the Belgian Village, a compound containing a few dozen beautiful, European-style homes built by the country's Belgian colonizers decades earlier. Many UN workers lived there, but it was not surrounded by a fence, and the UN troops guarding it were, in my estimation, not entirely reliable. The home I shared with two other Canadians had three bedrooms, but we all worked different shifts and had little interaction with one another. On several occasions I returned very late, when the other two men weren't home. Paranoid that someone might be lying in wait to kill me, I cleared the entire house room by room, pistol in hand, turning on all the lights to be certain I was alone. After doing that several times I remember lying in bed one night, with my pistol literally under my pillow, thinking how silly I was acting. "Why was I doing that?" I wondered.

My reaction to the death threat was not so much fear, but rather what is called hypervigilance. By the end of my tour this hypervigilance was so ingrained that I could not prevent myself from going through these same precautionary steps. A few nights after telling myself to "act normal," I arrived home at about 11:00 p.m. and once again found the lights off. I parked my jeep, took a deep breath, and reminded myself to relax when I went in. Although at the time I knew nothing about hypervigilance (I didn't even know the term existed), I knew I needed to regain control over my impulses, to bring back some kind of normalcy to my life. To this end, I walked confidently to the front door and put the key in the lock, but before I knew it I'd whipped my pistol out again, as if I was being controlled by some alien force. It felt almost like an addiction—I just couldn't stop myself from brandishing my weapon.

Once again, I went through the motions—turning on the lights, clearing the house, and falling asleep with the gun under my pillow.

SEVERAL WEEKS LATER, on a bright and sunny day in February 1995, I left UNHQ at noon for a meeting in downtown Kigali. Early in my drive I was pulled over by a Canadian military policeman for speeding. Given that several months earlier no one would have dared to suggest that a driver slow down—to do so would have made them an easy target for combatant forces—this seemed quite odd. During my time in Rwanda, driving had involved racing everywhere I went; being told I was speeding heralded another sign of how much things had changed since the beginning of my tour. Unfortunately, I hadn't changed along with them. Thankfully, though, the soldier was lenient about my heavy foot. We talked and joked for a few minutes, and then he let me continue my trip downtown without any penalty. The conversation nevertheless left me with a rather strange feeling about how quickly an environment can go from order to chaos and back again.

Driving into Kigali's downtown core involved negotiating a series of roundabouts. As I approached a large roundabout with four entry points I saw a large dump truck carrying over a dozen armed soldiers coming from the entry point across from me. The men inside were cheering, chanting, and evidently enjoying their day. Given the vehicle's size I decided it was best to let it enter the roundabout before me, so I stopped and watched it enter. It was immediately clear that the driver was moving quite fast, and as he entered the circle I could see the vehicle tip slightly to one side. The tires skidded as the truck built up a bit of speed, which caused the soldiers in the back to briefly stop their chanting and duck. A second later the driver regained control, but I had the premonition that something bad was about to happen. And indeed, instead of learning his lesson, the driver started accelerating again. I watched from across the way while wondering to myself, "What the hell is he doing?"

When the driver approached the second curve (to my left) I worried that he might hit me as he left the roundabout. I put my jeep in reverse in case I had to back up, and then waited. A few seconds later, as he passed by me on his way to the next turnoff, I could see that the truck was leaning again, this time at a sharper angle than before. Suddenly, it tipped over completely, sending the soldiers in all directions. As it was falling over I saw one man, who must've foreseen the accident, quickly climb over the back and leap out toward the ground. When he landed a few dozen feet to my right his head cracked open on the pavement.

I put the jeep in park. My first instinct was to get out and help the soldiers, many of whom were now bleeding on the pavement. But I was at my tipping point. I was tired of human tragedy, misery, and blood—I just couldn't do it anymore. I pondered over what to do, but after a few moments I decided, "The hell with this." Picking up my radio, I called it in to UNHQ and drove off. Sadly, I didn't even feel guilty about leaving the scene. My choice was irresponsible, certainly, some might even say reprehensible. But after so many months of witnessing bloodshed and destruction I just couldn't cope with another violent situation. This was yet another sign that my mind had reached a new and darker place. I should have felt guilty, but I didn't.

BY THIS POINT I'd been in Rwanda for nine months. UNHQ was now full of civilians—UN workers, expats from all over the world, and locally hired Rwandans. One day I noticed a beautiful black woman working as an administrative assistant in the central office, where photocopies and other paperwork were done. I noticed from the sound of her accent that she was Rwandan. She was dressed very nicely, and she carried herself with a certain aura of grace and elegance, like a movie star from Hollywood's golden age. I had been away from home for quite a while, and perhaps noticed her more than I would have under normal circumstances. After I'd visited the office a few times she happened to serve me at the front desk. The office was particularly busy that day, so after she helped me I carried on with my day's work.

A few days later I was walking down the hall as she approached from the opposite direction. When we got close we both said hello, and then she asked me where I was from. She lamented the fact that Valentine's Day was just around the corner but she didn't have a valentine. Then she looked me in the eye and asked if I would be her valentine. I was slightly taken aback. I always wore my wedding ring on deployments, so I assumed it was obvious I was unavailable. Feeling a little awkward and unsure of how to respond, I joked that I was taken but would be happy to meet her for a friendly coffee and chat. She laughed and we agreed to meet later that afternoon. If I'm being honest, I was certainly happy to converse with a beautiful woman for an hour or so, but more than that, I longed for any kind of friendship with someone outside the military. Throughout my tour I rarely spoke with civilians for longer than a few minutes, and even then usually about UN-related business. I was looking forward to a casual, friendly chat about life.

Over coffee we talked for quite a while. She seemed like a kind person. I learned during our conversation that she was a Tutsi who during the genocide hid from the Interahamwe, and even from some of her neighbours who sympathized with them. Although she survived, many of her family members were killed—sadly, a common story throughout the country. She was highly educated and well spoken. Somehow these qualities seemed to symbolize a different side of Rwanda, one I had seen only rare glimpses of during the war.

After an hour of chatting she mentioned that she knew of a Valentine's Day dinner being held at a club located at the top of the Belgian Village. She asked if I was interested in going. I was never one to enjoy big crowds, and I enjoyed them even less after the things I'd experienced in the past year, but no harm had come from our chat, so I agreed. We arranged for me to pick her up at her home, which happened to be located on the long back road leading to the airport.

A few days later I picked her up at her house and we drove to the Belgian Village. Once again she looked elegant, this time in a beautiful, brightly-coloured dress. We had a nice dinner and spoke with various UN personnel and other acquaintances. It felt strange and somehow wrong to be enjoying any kind of festivities in a country that had just been at war with itself, but I guess its citizens (and UN staff) needed events like this to get people's spirits up again.

At about 9:00, when people started trickling out of the restaurant, things became a bit awkward between us. She asked if I wanted to go somewhere else. My house, which was close by, had a nice patio, so we drove there and chatted about all sorts of things over a glass of wine. Suddenly the moment arrived that I, naive as I was, should've seen coming. She took my hand and placed it on her breast, at the same time reaching over and kissing me. I hadn't been intimate with my wife in almost a year, and I felt lonely and isolated. I'm not making excuses for my behaviour, but in hindsight I know just how much my morals and values were compromised by my experiences away from home. Instead of pushing her away I allowed it to happen.

Then, after a few moments, the gravity of the situation hit me like a ton of bricks. I pulled away and said, "I'm sorry, I can't do this." Though she looked dismayed, she said she understood. But then she turned her head away, looked down at the ground, and started to cry. I knew it had been far too short a time for her to really care about me, but she had been through a terrible ordeal; perhaps she just wanted some intimacy after experiencing so much misery and suffering. Under normal circumstances I don't think either of us would have put ourselves in this position, but the maelstrom of the last year affected all those caught up in it. With hindsight, I can certainly say that the night's events were yet another sign I'd reached my tipping point. Things I could never, ever have seen myself doing prior to my tour, like naively meeting up with a woman for coffee and dinner, now bypassed the area of my mind that previously would've prevented me from entering such situations.

I apologized to her again; that seemed like the only appropriate thing to do after turning down her advances. She reiterated that she understood, and we both leaned back in our chairs. We continued to chat for a few more minutes, and when I could see she had regained her composure I decided it was time to end the evening. The drive back to her house was less awkward than I expected, and we parted on amicable terms. Maybe we had a silent understanding that life was strange and surreal after the war, that we'd both acted out of character. Throughout the remainder of my tour we encountered each other numerous times in the hallways of UNHQ, and we always said hello to one another. Just before I left she was transferred to another office and I never saw her again. Sadly, with the passage of years I can't even remember her name.

IN MARCH THE time finally came for me to return home. The signal regiment had already returned in January, but since I was working directly for the UN I stayed on for a few more months to finish up some minor tasks. My later departure meant I would be flying home alone on a civilian airline rather than with my comrades on a military aircraft.

I spent the last several weeks helping my replacement learn the job and ensuring that my paperwork was in order. UN bureaucrats were having a hard time finding me a ticket from Kenya to Ottawa, which angered me because by March I was physically and mentally exhausted and couldn't wait to get back. I eventually grew impatient and began shopping around myself. I soon found a ticket from Nairobi to Ottawa that cost $1,600 and would let me leave in a week. For some nonsensical reason I can't recall (probably something to do with protocol), that arrangement didn't work for the UN, so I was stuck waiting. I bided my time by keeping busy and daydreaming about seeing my wife and kids. A few days later I got a call that they had finally found me something. I was summoned to come and sign for it, and when I saw the price my

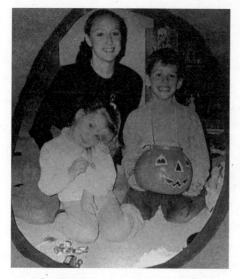

Julie, Veronique, and David, Hallow-
een 1994: Julie sent this family photo
to me while I was in Rwanda.

jaw dropped: $3,600 for a coach ticket. I guess they thought the extra $2,000 was no big deal.

The following week I caught a Hercules flight from Kigali to Nairobi, where I had to stay overnight. I arose early the next morning, put on civilian clothes, and went to the airport, boarding my flight without any difficulty. I was finally on my way home. Between my flight to London, where I had a four-hour layover, and then flights to Toronto and ultimately Ottawa, I had plenty of time to think back on my experiences over the past year.

Although it's been more than twenty years since I returned from Rwanda, I still vividly remember the thoughts and feelings I experienced on that journey home. The most prominent feeling was one of anticlimax. After witnessing and experiencing so much over the past ten months, I could now only mull over these memories in my head. I felt like I'd lived ten lifetimes, and yet I had no one to share these experiences with. Of course, I also felt relief and excitement that I was getting back to my family and home. But with this excitement came anxiety, especially over how I would reconnect with my wife Julie, my kids David and Veronique, and my old life. This was before the Internet and cell phones became common parts of daily life, and my sense of having been disconnected from home was profound.

Home and family life was, in a way, like a food I'd eaten a long time ago: I could remember eating it but I'd forgotten the nuances of how it tasted. This was, I imagine, a form of what travelers sometimes call reverse culture shock, though in my case that shock was mixed with memories of violence and bloodshed. When you've been gone almost a year and have lived in an entirely foreign environment, you also forget how things work at home. Rwanda had been my whole life. And in spite of the difficulties I'd experienced there, my needs were simple: do my job and stay alive. Essentially I had only to think about myself.

At home my responsibilities would be much larger and more diverse, and they were compounded, of course, by the realization that my tour had thrust all of these

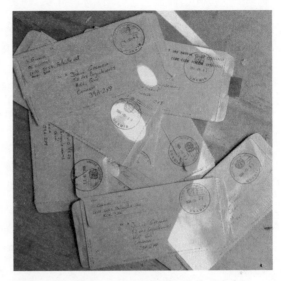

Some of the letters I sent to Julie while I was on the mission in Rwanda.

on Julie. She even had the immense stress of seeing the terrifying news each day and getting letters from my parents asking if she'd heard from me. I could only imagine what it would be like, both physically and emotionally, to suddenly have me thrust back into her life again. She would no doubt be happy to have me back, but life takes on its own rhythm when you're away, and I knew that she would have to adjust to what it was like to have her husband back in her life after almost a year of doing things on her own.

As the plane soared over Africa I was struck by the continent's immensity and grandeur. I remember leaning against the plane's fuselage as I looked out the window at the Sahara Desert. Ahead of the plane, as far as the eye could see, there was sand; I looked to my right at the tail of the plane, and below it was all sand, too. Africa's scenery and size were always breathtaking.

But a few memories continually occupied my mind as I made my way back to Canada. I remembered meeting a European agricultural specialist back in December, and the interesting conversation we'd had. He explained that in spite of its miniscule size, Rwanda had the potential to feed a very high percentage of the entire continent, if only its lands were used efficiently and saved from the ravages of war.

Thinking about that conversation as I flew over Africa caused me to wonder about potential solutions to the many problems its nations faced, some of which I'd witnessed firsthand.

I also recalled the extensive research I did in the lead-up to my tour, particularly about Rwanda's history and demographics. At the time I'd read an almanac that described the country's fertility rate as one of the highest in the world—almost 6.5 children per woman. Now, as we flew through the sky I couldn't believe how many Rwandans, human beings, had been tragically lost: 800,000 people—gone.

That thought now connected with an unnerving memory of one of my earliest days in Rwanda. I'd visited the King Faisal Hospital in Kigali a few days after I arrived, right in the midst of the civil war. At that time the hospital was occupied by doctors from the International Red Cross. Footage of that day shot by John Blouin is now with the Department of National Defence, most likely in an archive somewhere. When we showed up to check on the hospital and its staff the first thing we saw were women washing surgical gloves, intravenous tubes, and saline bags in the river. The river was far from clean, to say the least. When they finished with the washing they hung everything on clothes lines for the next day's rounds of surgery. Any tools were put on tarps and dried in the sun.

When we went inside, the situation was far worse. Piercing screams filled the halls. A man was having the dressings removed from his recently amputated leg, but they were stuck in place with coagulated blood. He was obviously in a tremendous amount of pain, but doctors didn't have the drugs to ease his suffering. I could only imagine the sensations shooting through his body. The doctors were visibly upset, especially when they told us that during the previous night the Interahamwe had come in and murdered a few people right in front of them. It took only a few days in Rwanda for me to be exposed to that sort of sadness and carnage. Now, as we flew over the continent, I took solace in the fact that I was finally leaving all of this behind—or so I thought.

Later, as the plane flew beyond Africa, I experienced a feeling of gratitude. Somehow I'd not been significantly injured. In fact, no visible damage had been done to me at all. For the first time it really dawned on me how lucky I was. Ten and a half months in one of the most chaotic places on the planet, and here I was, still in one piece. My mind then drifted back to the hospital in Kigali; I remembered looking at the surgical gloves being washed by the river and thinking, "I'd better not get shot here." In fact, after seeing the hospital's cleaning methods I was less afraid of being shot than I was of contracting some horrendous disease from the care I would receive.

Trying to process the multitude of factors that led to the many things I witnessed in Rwanda would challenge even the sturdiest moral compass. As human beings we live our lives generally understanding the difference between right and wrong, good and bad. You follow that compass your whole life, using it to make decisions and guide you on your path. Occasionally it leads you astray, but for the most part you can be certain it will take you where you need to go. When people experience extremely intense moments it's like a magnet has been held to their compass, shaking the very foundation of how it works and pulling them in all directions. If the magnet is only applied once and quickly removed the compass will return to working order without any serious problems. But if the magnet is held there repeatedly the compass will become permanently de-calibrated, never knowing which direction is magnetic north. As a Canadian who was brought up with very specific ideas of right and wrong, what I witnessed clashed with everything I thought I knew. What I experienced was a very slow, methodical de-calibration of my moral compass. Simplistic ideas about good and evil no longer applied.

Even when I wasn't consciously drawing on such concepts I now know that *unconsciously*, in the abyss of my mind, part of me was trying to process what these experiences meant. It wasn't trauma in the purest sense—it was more of a moral injury, a de-calibration of what I knew about the world and how it worked. Psychiatrists often misunderstand and underestimate the *moral conflict* that lies at the centre of "traumatic" events. If we don't try to understand these conflicts, we will never gain a full picture of the slow, insidious demise of the mind that is, in many ways, more difficult to deal with than pure "trauma." By the end of my Rwanda tour, the moral conflict I'd undergone had led me to a dark place, one in which I no longer cared about risk, danger, or death.

As the plane's engines hummed, these thoughts floated in and out of my head. I felt extremely lucky to be alive, but at the same time I sensed that something was lurking deep down inside of me. I knew I wasn't the Stéphane who'd left for Rwanda the previous year. I was irrevocably changed, I was sure, even if I couldn't figure out in what ways. But I tried to put these thoughts aside and think only about a happy future. What else could I do?

With Africa out of sight the plane continued toward London. I now felt fatigue and exhaustion setting in. I decided to try and get some sleep. I still had a long journey ahead of me.

Chapter 4

RETURNING HOME

I landed in Ottawa around dinnertime. I had only a few more hurdles to clear before taking a cab home.

The first was retrieving my luggage. While I stood waiting at the baggage carousel I looked around at all of the people pushing and jockeying for position, many in a rush to snatch their luggage and get out of the airport a few seconds earlier than the person beside them. Outwardly I was calm, but inside my blood boiled with frustration, resentment, and pent-up anger. I had been away for almost a year, and had witnessed some of the worst humanity had to offer—"What the hell are *these people* in a rush for?" I wondered. What kind of hardships had these insensitive fools experienced? Of course, they had no way of knowing where I'd been or what I'd seen, but that didn't enter my mind. All I felt was bitterness and anger. Unbeknownst to me, these thoughts were a sign that a rift was already forming between myself and the society in which I lived. After standing and watching the strange, quasi-animalistic behaviour of my fellow passengers I saw my bags slide onto the carousel. I waded through the crowd and grabbed them, ready to get away from what I thought was the source of my anger. I took a deep breath as I put my luggage on a cart and thought, "Well, I guess I'm home."

Toward the end of my time in Rwanda my return had been delayed or cancelled numerous times, which always disappointed Julie and the kids. Since I was unsure right up until the last minute that this would indeed be my actual return date, I'd avoided telling anyone. Instead, I decided I would just fly home unannounced, catch a cab, and surprise them at the front door. So I made my way to the taxi stand—where I again had to stand in line. I could feel my blood pressure beginning to rise, just as it had at the luggage carousel. All I wanted was to get home, and even these simple hurdles seemed unusually frustrating and difficult. Thankfully, in very little time I was in a taxi and on the way home.

At the time—March 1995—we were living in Hull, Quebec, a short trip across the Champlain Bridge from Ottawa, but because I'd arrived at the tail end of rush hour the ride from the airport took about forty minutes. I was in a dream-like state and avoided conversation with the driver. I was mostly afraid of him asking me where I'd arrived from, of having to either tell him the truth or make up a story. The last thing I wanted was to get into a conversation with a stranger about Rwanda. What would I say? "Oh yeah, it's pretty bad there." Thankfully, he seemed to sense that I was not in a talkative mood, and after initial pleasantries we shared a comfortable silence. I slouched in my seat and stared out the window, wondering how my family would receive me.

The cab pulled up at about 7:30 p.m. I got out, paid the driver, and stood for a moment, admiring our little row house. I was finally home. I could see the kids' bedroom lights on upstairs; it looked like everyone was still awake. I walked slowly up the steps leading to the front door and paused for a moment. I never brought a house key with me overseas, since there were numerous opportunities for it to get lost, so I had no way of unlocking the door. Instead I pushed the doorbell and waited in anticipation. I heard the muffled sound of movement inside as Julie made her way to the door, with the kids not far behind, wondering who was ringing at that hour of the day. A few seconds later the door slowly opened and there was Julie, with the kids right behind her. She was happily surprised; Veronique and David looked a little shocked. They weren't expecting me, and were perhaps a little unsure that the man at the front door was indeed their dad. Like all kids dealing with mixed emotions, they were uncertain of what to do. Seeing the slight confusion on their faces, I said hello as cheerfully as I could and stepped inside.

As soon as my feet touched the doormat I was completely over-whelmed with emotion. The kids were now rushing toward me, and as I bent down to hug them I fell on my knees. It felt as though all of the blood had rushed out of my head and my energy had been totally sapped. A range of thoughts and feelings rushed through my brain: Rwanda, home; home, Rwanda. Luckily, the impact of my knees hit-ting the ground, combined with the kids hugging me, snapped me out of it and I regained control.

Outwardly, the timing of my fall had made it appear intentional, but as I hugged the children and then Julie I knew something very unusual had occurred. That fainting episode (for lack of a better description) would stay with me, and years later, when I became an advisor to the military on operational stress injuries, this memory would lead me to delve into the literature on soldiers' homecoming transition. It was clear from my own experience, and that of many other soldiers during the 1990s, that the military needed to prevent soldiers from going from the regimented and sometimes harrowing environment of deployment to the tranquil and happy environment of "home" without any sort of interim adjustment period.

ALMOST INVARIABLY, WHEN a soldier first returns from a long overseas deployment, things are at first cheery and positive. After being away from family, dealing with distressing events, experiencing intense cul-ture shock, and lacking many creature comforts, soldiers are happy just to be home. Health concerns, especially mental ones, usually fall pretty low on the priority list during that initial period of euphoria. Some sol-diers with mental health problems crash shortly after this honeymoon phase is over, but I was able to get back into a routine relatively quickly, which somewhat helped to ease my transition and keep me going.

And yet, shortly after my return I started to undergo some changes. It wasn't any single event that signalled this transition, but rather various subtle shifts that, in retrospect, acted as signs of things to come. In April I returned to the National Defence Media Liaison Office (MLO) and resumed my pre-Rwanda job as a media liaison officer. One day shortly thereafter I received a call from the military logistics staff telling me my equipment from Rwanda had arrived in Ottawa. I promptly drove to the airport, signed for it, and brought it back home.

The following weekend was unusually sunny and warm for that time of year, so I decided to open up my barracks boxes and equipment bags, and clean and sort through things in the driveway. As I began my work, Veronique was happily taking advantage of the good weather to ride her tricycle around on our dead-end street. After watching her enjoy herself for a few minutes I opened everything up, attached the hose, and began by cleaning my boots. I picked one up and began spraying the sole, which still had Rwandan soil stuck in it. Just then Veronique started walking up the driveway with a curious look on her face, to see what I was doing. With the juxtaposition of these two sights—my daughter approaching while the red soil washed down the driveway—I suddenly panicked. The idea of my daughter and the Rwandan soil being in close proximity to each other symbolized the coming together of two worlds that had to be kept apart, and I was horrified at the thought of my daughter getting even a drop of that tainted soil on her. There were so many thoughts and images going through my head at that moment that I reacted without thinking. In a curt and authoritative tone I told her to get back on her tricycle and go up toward the house.

I was so focused on spraying those boots and washing away all that red soil—an act of symbolic cleansing—that the gentle father in me had momentarily fled. In another state of mind I would've been much kinder, would've just picked Veronique up, put her back on her tricycle, and sent her on her way. Outwardly, the event wasn't anything intensely dramatic: anyone watching might have just thought I was in a bad mood. But inwardly, a chasm was already forming between myself and the "normal" people around me. Together with other, similar events, this incident demonstrated that I was sliding down a slippery slope toward a mental break. The problem was I just wasn't watching out for it.

As the weeks passed, nights became increasingly difficult. I was very restless, had numerous nightmares, and often had trouble sleeping. Days weren't much better. Julie noticed me becoming increasingly impatient, flying off the handle over very slight inconveniences or setbacks. Losing sleep, being tormented by my dreams, and starting my days upset and emotional created a domino effect that impacted my whole social world. I was also very confused. Where, I wondered, did these feelings originate? Did the lack of sleep lead to nightmares, or did the nightmares lead to lack of sleep? Where did Rwanda fit into all of this? Was I just experiencing a temporary rough period? Untangling cause and effect wasn't easy—even in retrospect it's tough to sort out these initial experiences. But one thing was clear: my inner core was gradually being altered by the perfect storm brewing inside me—the swirl of emotions, memories of Rwanda, and my recent transition to home and normality.

As the fall approached, things became extremely hectic at NDHQ. At that time, the Belgian government was coming down really hard on General Dallaire for the death in Rwanda of ten Belgian soldiers under his command. They essentially wanted him brought to Europe for questioning. The UN, for its part, refused to send him. My bosses at NDHQ were asked to help, and since I'd served under Dallaire in Rwanda, I was sent to Montreal along with two others to help him with his response to the Belgian government's questions. This was a busy time to say the least.

During this period I worked a lot of evenings, but one day I decided to go home for dinner and eat with the family; I'd have to return to work and finish up later on, but a bit of time at home seemed like a welcome respite. So I drove home, had a nice meal with Julie and the kids, and shortly after headed back to finish my tasks. My mind felt like it was operating normally, but then something strange and unsettling happened: out of nowhere, while driving back to NDHQ, I had a sudden and very strong impulse to wrap my car around a telephone pole.

I was coming down a hill near the University of Quebec, and as the car built up speed I thought, "I'm going to wrap my car around a pole. That's it, I'm done." The idea came in a flash. I had never even thought of the word *suicide* before—it just wasn't in my vocabulary. And yet here I was, with the overwhelming desire to drive at high speed into a pole. Luckily, the thought quickly disappeared. It was then that the gravity of the situation hit home. I thought, "What the hell am I doing?" It was quite disturbing, the way this destructive thought had arrived without warning and then just as suddenly vanished.

I tried to put this scare out of my mind, and I didn't tell Julie about it when I got home later that night. But the next morning, as I put on my uniform and prepared to head back to work, I was consumed by thoughts of what might have happened. I had a beautiful wife, two great kids, and a good job. Everything seemed fine. I just couldn't figure out what was wrong. Although many soldiers felt—and still feel—anxious about seeing a doctor for psychiatric difficulties, largely due to the stigma around mental health in the military, I didn't even know what stigma was. And so, instead of going to work, I went to the National Defence Medical Centre (NDMC) in Ottawa. It wasn't the norm at that time for a soldier to seek medical attention so soon after a deployment for mental health issues, but I didn't really think about it, I just went.

When I got to the parking lot at the NDMC, *that* was when the notion of stigma started to kick in. After parking the car I had to go to what we in the military call "sick parade," a dedicated time each day when soldiers can report to a doctor. I knew that when I went inside they were going to ask me to fill out a form with all my information and my reason for visiting. As I thought about the previous night I didn't know what I should write. I felt embarrassed. The person behind the front desk was usually a junior non-commissioned officer. I didn't have a big ego, but as a captain the thought of disclosing the fact that I was suicidal to a corporal was slightly humiliating. For about fifteen minutes I sat in the car and contemplated how I would handle things. Finally, I bucked myself up enough to go inside.

Like I expected, a master corporal greeted me at the front desk. We exchanged the customary greetings and he gave me a form. I filled it out but left the "reason for visit" box blank. When I returned the form the corporal quickly scanned it and told me I needed to fill in why I was there. I said that it was difficult to explain, that I just wanted to speak with a doctor. He politely repeated his request. My style of command was never based on bullying or browbeating my subordinates, but at that moment, with feelings of shame and embarrassment forefront in my mind, I just glared at him and said, "If you don't let me see a doctor without filling out this damned sheet of paper you're going to see me back here in a body bag."

Taken aback by my response, the corporal now understood it was necessary to sidestep protocol, and he allowed me to proceed without finishing the form. The whole waiting room had of course heard my outburst, and as I went to find a seat I felt embarrassed. I picked up a magazine and did my best to cover my face, but I knew those waiting were probably wondering what was wrong with me. I now felt both the stigma of asking for help and the shame of dressing down that poor corporal in front of the whole room. Minutes seemed like hours as I stared blankly at the magazine, waiting for my name to be called.

Within half an hour I was in front of a female physician. She listened attentively as I explained my situation, and because of her calm, gentle demeanour I felt confident that she'd be able to fix me right up. But after about ten minutes she told me that she suspected I might have what she called "PTSD." Although I'd heard that term in passing a few times I had no idea what it meant. She concluded our appointment by saying that my malady was beyond her expertise and that she was referring me to a specialist. A week later I had an appointment with a military psychiatrist.

I saw that psychiatrist (whose name I've omitted) three or four times over the course of about six weeks. On the first visit, he greeted me and mentioned that he had a nursing student doing her practicum in mental health care; as long as I didn't mind, she would attend our first session, and perhaps future ones as well. I didn't know what to say, so I just agreed. All I can remember from my sessions with him are very in-depth, if somewhat mundane, analytical questions: "How's your life? Do you have any debts? What was your childhood like?"— that sort of thing. This line of questioning sounded to me like something from a Woody Allen movie, and I felt it didn't really get to the heart of anything. I was a veteran of Rwanda, a country that had seen some of the worst atrocities since the Second World War, and all he could ask me about was my childhood. I had greater concerns, like figuring out what was keeping me up at night, why I had collapsed in the doorway when I got home, and why I flipped out on my daughter that day in the driveway. I knew nothing about psychiatry or psychology, but I was certain my difficulties weren't because of a bad childhood or my relationship with my father.

I therefore left my first appointment feeling disillusioned. But I understood that Rome wasn't built in a day, as the saying goes, so I decided to allow time for the process to work. But the second appointment was the same, and then the third, and eventually I was prescribed a bunch of pills. At that point I was tempted to give up. Right from the get-go there was no therapeutic alliance, which is to say, there was no connection or engagement between us; I was just another patient being given the one-size-fits-all remedy of talk therapy and pills. He might have been a competent clinician, but he appeared to have no people skills and didn't understand how to get to the root of what troubled me. People knew what happened in Rwanda—why was he asking me about my childhood and how my father treated me? We weren't talking about what *I* thought was disturbing me; instead we were talking about what *he* wanted to discuss. I went home with very little understanding of even what the pills he prescribed were for. Simply put, I had no confidence in him or his ability to help me. Later I flushed the pills down the toilet. I never went to see him as a patient again. And in fact, by a twist of fate, down the road he became somewhat of a nemesis as I tried to change the military's mental health system.

Like numerous soldiers during the 1990s, I'd come into contact with a dysfunctional military health-care system and stale psychiatric methods, not to mention many doctors who were unaware of what war and peacekeeping could do to a person's mind. The military was completely unprepared to deal with the aftermath of sending thousands of people on peacekeeping missions that involved no peace at all. My initial experiences after seeking help inspired me to try and change what was evidently a broken and archaic system.

THE MID-1990S WERE trying years for the Canadian military, which was engaged in several active peacekeeping operations across the globe. The Cold War had recently ended and the world was dealing with the fallout of wars caused by the power vacuum opened by the collapse of the Soviet Union in 1991. My workplace, the MLO, was the hub of communications for the entire Department of National Defence (DND), including for those units stationed overseas. On the list of daily issues to be dealt with there was the constant turmoil in the Balkans, the inquiry into the murder of Somalis at the hands of members of the Canadian Airborne Regiment in 1993 (the so-called Somalia Affair), and of course the fallout from the mission to Rwanda. At times it seemed like there was a new controversy every week, but on top of work stresses I was slowly falling apart. Over time, I was learning, mental erosion can be as damaging as any physical injury.

In October 1996 the *Vancouver Province* published photos taken by Canadian military engineers in Kuwait during the Gulf War. In some of the photos the engineers were posed beside the body parts of dead Iraqi soldiers, and in some cases they were shown smiling or appearing to clown around. The story was quickly picked up by the *Toronto Star* and other major newspapers across the country, further stoking the already stressful situation created by the Somalia Affair. Under a great deal of public pressure the minister of national defence, Doug Young, denounced the combat engineers' actions, stating that he didn't think much of those who took pictures beside bodies. An investigation was ordered, but rumours abounded that the soldiers involved might be released.

I was flabbergasted by the reactions of both politicians and members of the public to this event. I had pictures of myself with dead bodies in Rwanda, as did many others, though I never treated the situation with levity. What the minister and the public failed to understand was that experiencing such a surreal moment for the first time often caused soldiers to want to document the event, and sometimes to use a tasteless but timeless defence mechanism—dark humour—to deflect their real feelings about witnessing traumatic sights. Their actions were definitely in bad taste by normal, peacetime standards, and they deserved some kind of censure, but they didn't deserve to be pilloried the way they were, or released from the military. Soldiers take photos in those situations for many reasons. In the Balkans, for example, some Canadian peacekeepers had taken personal photos of genocide victims, often simply to deny perpetrators the chance to say it never happened.* For others, photography was a chance to capture the event, to remind themselves that it wasn't just a nightmare, that it really did happen. The minister of defence and other politicians had turned on soldiers who'd done a very difficult and dangerous job in the Middle East simply to deflect criticism. Put simply, the tasteless behaviour in some of the photos was wrong, but taking photos was not.

My colleague, Alain Ouellette, and I were both completely floored when hearing those at the DND, many of whom had never gotten their boots dirty, give their misinformed and naive interpretation of how the psyche reacts in these types of situations. After talking it over, we decided to call the journalists Jocelyn Coulon and David Pugliese, at *Le Devoir* and the *Ottawa Citizen*, respectively. Coulon conducted an interview with Alain and me that weekend, and Pugliese later came to my house for a two-hour chat.

We showed them pictures we had of ourselves with bodies and stated that if the minister was going to fire Canadian military engineers he would have to fire us, too, because we had similar photos (though minus any instances of joking around). Put simply, we went public and came to our fellow soldiers' defence. Given that the military and the DND never like soldiers speaking to the media, we knew

---

*   Readers looking to know more about this phenomenon should read journalist Carol Off's 2004 book *The Ghosts of Medak Pocket: The Story of Canada's Secret War.*

our actions would be met with disapproval; technically, we hadn't even been given permission to do what we did. So we wrote a memo to our boss, a colonel, informing him of our rationale and providing justification for our actions. Unfortunately, by that point the issue was already highly politicized, and the chain of command had done what it tended to do in situations like this: kowtow to the minister of defence.

On Monday morning the colonel found two things on his desk: our memo and articles from *Le Devoir* and the *Ottawa Citizen*. He was absolutely livid, while the minister, for his part, wanted our heads. The next month was therefore very tough. We kept doing our jobs, but we knew there would be some sort of consequences. And indeed, a month later we were eventually pulled into our commandant's office to sign a "report of shortcomings," which warned us that we had six months to correct our behaviour or else face release from the military.

In my case, the chain of command knew I was having some difficulty after my time in Rwanda, but still they chose a punitive tack. They strongly suggested that I see a psychiatrist, and informed me that if I didn't sort myself out in six months they would kick me out. Of course, they weren't entirely wrong that I needed help—I certainly wasn't doing well. But I hadn't challenged the DND and the military's chain of command simply because of my mental state. Perhaps I went further than I normally would have in these circumstances, but I would have taken action to show solidarity with my comrades no matter what.

At any rate, I now had six months to get a clean bill of health, or else I would get the boot. As a young captain with a wife, two kids, and a mortgage, I needed to keep my career, which meant I had to heed the chain of command's "suggestion." Shortly thereafter I was referred to a psychologist. Over the many weeks that I saw her I kept any mention of nightmares, anxiety attacks, or cold sweats to myself—so concerned was I with showing my superiors a clean bill of health. In the end, my ruse worked: I was given a passing grade and I was allowed to continue my job. The report of shortcomings was removed from my file, and I carried on.

Years later, in 2008–09, I was working with a social worker and friend, Suzanne Bailey, whom I'd met through the National Speakers Bureau, an organization that brings a wide range of Canadian thought leaders to conferences around the country. Suzanne told me of a conversation she'd had with my psychologist, who said she knew I'd been lying during our sessions together.* She had been unsure of how to respond: she knew I wasn't well, but she also sensed that I was in a tough spot in terms of my career. Unknowingly, I'd caused her to become engaged in a moral and ethical conflict over whether to help me salvage my career or call my bluff and potentially cause my release from the military, with all the consequences such an outcome would entail. Mental health challenges, as I was to learn, affect not just the patient, but the professional, too.

My lying was another example of the odd and irrational behaviour that found its way into my life after Rwanda. Survival was my number one goal, and I was prepared to lie, even about my own health, to ensure that I achieved it. And yet my job—the very thing on which I pinned my hopes of survival—was not without its harmful effects. Researchers now know that added stress, along with a lack of social support, in the wake of trauma is one of the major risk factors in the development of PTSD. My job at the communications office was a hectic and stressful one, and I have often wondered whether or not my mental state would have sunk so low if I'd returned to a more cushy job instead. There will never be a definite answer to that question, but I suspect that the stress certainly added fuel to the fire that was already burning inside me.

ALAIN AND I had met way back in 1984. As an officer cadet I had been sent to do my Canadian Airborne Regiment parachute course in Edmonton that year. When I arrived I shared sleeping quarters with four

---

* I realize that this sounds like my psychologist acted very unprofessionally, but at that point we were all good friends, and I'd discussed it openly with them both, so there was no breach of confidentiality.

other guys, one of whom was Alain. At the time he was a lieutenant. The course, which was tough but exhilarating for a young guy, lasted three weeks. Throughout that time Alain and I hit it off nicely, and we ended up spending lots of time together during the few free hours we had after our daily training. After the course was finished I was sent back to armoured school in Gagetown, New Brunswick, to continue my training as a troop leader in the armoured regiment. Alain went back to the Royal Twenty-second Regiment in Quebec, where he was already serving as a fully trained infantry officer.

I was beginning to think that I'd never get a chance to test the skills I had learned over the past several years: the Gulf War had come and gone, and the Canadian military hadn't seen any action. In 1992 I therefore requested a transfer to public relations at the MLO. My request was promptly accepted and, after a brief stint at Ryerson University, I started my new position. Though I didn't know it at the time, Alain, who'd chosen to change courses, would be posted to the MLO in 1995: one morning I showed up and, to my surprise, there he was. Before that, in 1992, Alain and the First Battalion of the Royal Twenty-second Regiment had been sent to Bosnia-Herzegovina as part of the Canadian peacekeeping force. They were the first Canadian peacekeepers added to the United Nations Protection Force there, which was created to help restore peace in the Balkans after the Cold War ended and the former Yugoslavia collapsed.* Peacekeepers like Alain who participated in those early days witnessed some of the most horrific things human beings can do to one another.

By 1995, when Alain began work at the MLO, over ten years had elapsed since our parachute course, but we had fond memories of each other and we reconnected easily. Within a short time we were having lunches together and our families were enjoying barbecues at each other's homes. And yet I was unaware that he, too, was experiencing

---

* In addition to Carol Off's *The Ghosts of Medak Pocket*, I highly recommend Jocelyn Coulon's *Soldiers of Diplomacy: The United Nations, Peacekeeping, and the New World Order*, for anyone looking to know more about what Canadian peacekeepers dealt with in the 1990s.

emotional difficulties dealing with the fallout from his deployment in the Balkans. I now wonder how many hundreds or thousands of others kept quiet about their health issues throughout this period. Of course, we will probably never know.

One day in the fall of 1995 Alain and I were alone in the office enjoying a short respite from the usual cacophony of our jobs. During the time we'd spent together he'd frequently seen me anxious and very irritable; he could see I was unwell. Gradually, he started asking questions about how things were going at home, how I was doing, and whether I was getting enough sleep. That day I answered him in short, clipped sentences, claiming that everything was fine. In the weeks that followed, though, I slowly became more comfortable answering his questions in a more open and honest manner. Very naturally our conversations morphed from friendly chats to true peer support. Without even knowing it, for the first time in my life I was receiving a natural, non-clinical type of support that allowed me to express my concerns and relieve my burden.

I'll always remember one such conversation, which took place a week later. I arrived at work looking haggard, and my mood matched my appearance. Just a few minutes into the day I was snapping at colleagues and acting irritable with anyone who dared to approach me. Then Alain walked over. At first, he gently informed me that I didn't look well. I quickly told him to fuck off, and said that I was fine. He stood at my desk and calmly but firmly said, "Stop being a jerk."

Alain understood that Rwanda had been tough for me, just as his time in the Balkans had been. Over the next several minutes he related a story from his time in Bosnia, when he stumbled upon a bucket containing three human heads. Then he opened up even further. He told me that he'd been to see a doctor, and said I should consider doing the same. Anybody who has ever felt the sharp sword of stigma will know how courageous an admission that was for him to make. When the conversation finished he walked away while I remained at my desk, mulling over our exchange. Alain's honesty, both toward me and about his own situation, allowed me to see that it wasn't necessarily a bad thing to seek medical help for something I didn't understand.

At the time I felt medical help was only something to seek if I had a broken leg or a bad case of the flu. The fact that I was upset and losing sleep all the time just didn't strike me as reasons to go see a doctor. I wasn't trying to take the easy way out—I simply didn't know medical treatment was an option. Alain helped changed all that.

Society teaches us that certain events, whether happy or sad, are appropriate to discuss with colleagues and friends—the birth of a baby, for example, or the death of an elderly parent. Even though we may be slightly uncomfortable discussing the latter case, we at least know that death is something we can express our discomfort about. The trouble with mental health problems is that most people are uncomfortable discussing them. This difficulty is compounded by the fact that many people can't even tell when a friend or colleague has such a problem. Alain, by contrast, was very adroit at opening up the necessary type of conversation. His approach made me feel comfortable sharing a little more with him each time we talked. After hearing we had faced some mutual challenges from our time overseas, I felt I could relate to him, and vice versa. Those conversations were my first taste of peer support, and this proved to be a key moment in my life. I was now aware that it was acceptable to seek help. That first, simple connection, that tough love and authentic human exchange, was crucial. It was the first domino to fall, and it started a chain reaction that gradually brought me to a greater understanding of my own issues and the power of peer support.

THE SOMALIA AFFAIR continued to dominate discussions at NDHQ throughout 1995. The previous year a high-profile inquiry had been launched into the 1993 torture and murder of Somali teenager Shidane Arone at the hands of Canadian peacekeepers. Prior to that, in April 1993, Canadian news media broke the story that the DND had altered documents sought through access to information requests after Arone's death became public. Various versions of the same documents were accidentally sent out by defence officials, so it didn't take reporters long to discover something was afoot. The alterations had been done in the very office that I now worked in, further fanning the flames. The military and the DND were in hot water.

My colleagues and I at the MLO were on the front line, dealing with the crisis from a media-response standpoint. What that meant for me was that the moral conflicts I encountered in Rwanda on an almost daily basis were being followed by conflicts of a different sort here in Canada. We were told by our superiors to commit illegal acts, and I was often forced to choose between personal integrity and duty to the organization I served. Since document alterations had taken place under the auspices of our office, colleagues also began to divide themselves into clans, usually based on loyalty to those who had broken the law.

When Jean Boyle was appointed chief of the defence staff (i.e., head of the Canadian Armed Forces) he ordered all offices of the military and the DND to search for documents related to Somalia and turn them in, apparently in the spirit of transparency.* After some digging we found a slew of files, which we turned over for release to the media. Simultaneously, there was another media request pertaining to a soldier, Corporal Daniel Gunther, killed in Bosnia in June 1993. The official story was that Gunther died from shrapnel wounds when a mortar fell close to his armoured personnel carrier. Understandably, his family wanted to figure out *exactly* what happened. Given the ostensibly transparent air blowing through the office with the Somalia Affair in full swing, I was tasked with tracking down all documents related to Gunther's death.

While going through the files I noticed that one of the incident reports referred back to a previous report that was nowhere to be found. Our office's files were very well maintained, so my curiosity was immediately piqued when I learned of this missing document. After scouring the office I eventually found the missing report, which provided some damning details—namely, that shortly before Gun-

---

* The highest rank in the Canadian Forces is the governor general, the Queen's representative. Typically, though, the chief reports to the minister of national defence.

ther's death Serb forces had warned Canadian peacekeepers not to position their anti-tank missiles in a certain area. They cited the menacing appearance of such equipment, and threatened to shoot at any Canadian vehicle with anti-armour capabilities. In other words, the report made clear that Canadian forces had essentially played a game of chicken with local combatant forces; it also implied that Gunther's vehicle was hit with an anti-tank rocket of some sort and that his death was no accident. The truth was that Gunther himself was hit in the chest by the anti-tank rocket. Enemy forces had deliberately fired at him, and the rocket killed him instantly.

After discovering and reading the missing incident report I brought it back to the MLO so that it could be released to the media and Gunther's family. But, in contrast to what I thought was a new spirit of openness and transparency, some of my superiors' first reaction was to destroy it. The document wouldn't necessarily have cast Canadian commanders in a favourable light, since it implied that they had disregarded threats from Serb forces, causing a soldier's death.* But in the wake of the Somalia Affair it was necessary to be honest with the public. I was nonetheless told to shred the document, and indeed to deny I ever found it. When I refused, arguments ensued, and the office was divided even further between those who insisted on transparency and those who continued to follow the archaic instinct to doctor and destroy documents. I was flabbergasted that in the wake of the Somalia Affair some in the department still thought it prudent to disregard the law and try to avoid public scrutiny.

My stress was further heightened when a friend and colleague, Captain Joel Brayman, was summoned to testify at the Somalia inquiry. Our boss, whose name I will omit, was also putting pressure on a civilian secretary in our office, who herself later testified at the inquiry. One morning she approached me, Brayman, and Chris Henderson

---

*   It's difficult to question the motives of Canadian commanders on the ground, though. Oftentimes it is necessary for UN peacekeepers to demonstrate to combatant forces that they will not be intimidated or deterred from fulfilling their mandate.

(whom, as you'll recalled from chapter 1, I spoke with on the phone while in Rwanda), saying she needed to speak with someone; since we were three of the guys who'd shown some personal integrity, she felt safe asking our advice. We all met for a coffee one morning, and during our discussion the secretary told us that she was given orders to get rid of and alter files, which understandably made her very uncomfortable. Even more shocking, she told us that she feared for her safety. We listened with concern, but were at a loss for exactly what to do. The moral conflict raging inside my head grew as each day passed.

Months later, when Joel testified at the Somalia inquiry, he mentioned the secretary's claim of intimidation at the hands of her boss. Sadly, when it was her turn to testify, she completely denied that the intimidation had ever occurred. Perhaps she was scared about what telling the truth might do to her career or physical safety, but in the end that put Joel, and to a lesser degree Chris and me, in a kettle of boiling water.

Because we had disobeyed orders, for the next year and beyond we were sometimes targeted by colleagues. One morning, for example, I arrived at my cubicle to find the definition of loyalty printed out and sitting on my chair—a not-so-subtle way of reminding me that I hadn't played the game the way some of my colleagues wanted me to. Chris and I were particularly fearful of how such tension would affect our military careers. Over a coffee we decided to seek advice from a representative of the information commissioner of Canada.* The meeting went well, and afterward we got in touch with Michael McAuliffe from the CBC, the journalist who'd originally broken the story about the alteration of documents.

We met with Michael in a coffee shop at Ottawa's Sparks Street Mall and explained everything in grueling detail. Michael was very knowledgeable and understood how to put the squeeze on bureaucratic organizations. The three of us agreed that Michael would withhold the information we'd provided *unless* Chris or I were court-

---

* The information commissioner assists those who feel that federal agencies have not respected their rights under the Access to Information Act.

martialed for disobeying a lawful order, something we suspected might happen. This was a pre-emptive attempt to salvage our integrity and get our story out if we were trampled on by superiors.

While we sat with Michael, a guy with a trench coat and a moustache—he resembled Peter Sellers as Inspector Clouseau in *The Pink Panther* movies—listened from a table beside us. He ordered no coffee or drink, and seemed to be pretending to read the newspaper while constantly glancing over at us. Even more suspiciously, he chose to sit beside us despite the fact that the place was otherwise totally empty. In less than a minute we surmised that he was probably from the National Investigation Service (NIS), an arm of the Canadian Forces Military Police. I thought those guys were clueless at the best of times. Apparently, though, our paranoia was well founded.

After spilling the beans to Michael we went to see Ruth Cardinal, the director general of public affairs—our civilian boss at the DND (and the boss of the colonel who intimidated his secretary). We told her everything going on under her watch, as well as our recent actions to protect ourselves. She couldn't believe her ears. The chain of command often tried to keep their civilian bosses from discovering exactly what they were up to, so she had no idea about any of this. We asked her to do the right thing, which meant telling the top brass to start following the law. We also informed her in no uncertain terms that if we were punished Michael McAuliffe would break the story we gave him, shaming the Canadian Forces and the DND even further. After we finished she sat there for a moment, stunned. She then wrote a few things on a piece of paper, thanked us for the information, and did her best to act unsurprised as she concluded the meeting.

In the end, the only concrete action the DND took was to pull us in front of the NIS for interrogation. Ironically, one of the guys who came to pick me up was Inspector Clouseau, from the coffee shop. A few by-the-book types sat me down in a tiny room with a bright light and asked numerous questions while a camera looked on. I answered their questions but remained defiant. When it was over I left; nothing more came of the discussion.

Although I escaped with my career intact, the moral and ethical conflicts I went through during this period added another layer of stress to what was already a fraught personal situation. Rwanda was always in the back of my mind, which meant I was already engaged in a daily battle with my own inner demons. That battle was made even more difficult by my having to face constant worries about my career, and ostracism from my colleagues and former friends. In retrospect, I have no doubt that the secondary wounding I incurred during this period helped cause my unravelling. Had I come back to a normal job, steady routine, and proper social support, who knows what path my life might have taken?

IN THE FALL of 1996 I had the opportunity to take over a team of about a half-dozen people at NDHQ for a unique assignment. My task was to create a combat camera team that could rapidly deploy overseas and gather footage of military operations. Filming our operations was a way to let the Canadian public know what was happening with their troops—an important measure of transparency in the wake of the Somalia Affair and other scandals of the 1990s. Throughout the year I worked hard to keep preparations rolling, and by 1997 the team was ready. We had a lot of high-tech equipment and were able to deploy in a very short period of time. On the inside, of course, I often wanted to jump out of my skin, so I grasped at any chance to do a short deployment overseas: I saw this as a way of escaping my troubles. The numerous missions Canada was involved in throughout the 1990s provided me with many such chances, and between 1997 and 1999 I ended up deploying to a number of spots around the world. In this way I became addicted to the adrenalin high that such missions injected me with.

Cambodia was my first taste of action since Rwanda. The Cambodians had recently established a tentative peace after many brutal years of civil war and genocide. My team spent several weeks there in the winter of 1997 working with Lieutenant-Colonel Chip Bowness and the Canadian Mine Action Centre. Their goal was to teach Cambodians how to de-mine the country; our job was to film their efforts. I had never been to a place as busy and hectic as Cambodia. I was constantly amazed at Cambodians' ability to transport a man, his wife, their two children, a pig, and several crates—all on one little scooter. I was even more amazed at their ability to navigate the busy, narrow, and chaotic roads that always seemed to be covered with a layer of dried-up sludge. It was nice to find temporary relief from the stresses plaguing my mind, but the stifling heat and humidity made me look forward to my next deployment.

Over the next few years my team and I would go to Lebanon, Haiti, and the Persian Gulf. These missions, and the chance for travel and adventure that they brought, helped get me through a two-year period during which my mind was constantly on the brink of shutting down; but that high couldn't last forever.

BY 1998 GENERAL Dallaire had been made the military's assistant deputy minister of human resources. One morning he called and said he wanted to produce an informational video that would show what had happened to Canadian soldiers in Rwanda, and he asked me if I could take care of it. Although I wasn't in his immediate chain of command, we were still in semi-regular contact, so I met with him and accepted the task. After doing some initial research I discovered that we wouldn't be able to obtain funding for a purely historical video; there had to be some kind of training component to it. I met with General Dallaire again, told him the situation, and suggested we focus on the mission's psychological effects. By taking that tack we could still have a historical element but also sell it as a "lessons learned" sort of video. He liked the idea and told me to get started. The final outcome was a powerful video called *Witness the Evil*.

During the production process I contacted a number of colleagues who'd experienced difficult times in Rwanda and asked them if they would share what they had been through both during and after their deployments. To make the video I hired a company called Affinity Productions, whose owner Ron Gallant and producer Jamie Banks dedicated heart and soul to the project. They wrote a script and we conducted a series of gut-wrenching on-camera interviews with Canadian soldiers. But when I was asked to do an interview I declined; my task was to allow other soldiers to tell their stories, not to place myself in the limelight. Jamie nonetheless insisted that I appear in the video in *some* capacity, so after some discussion I agreed to be in a short introductory scene. A young man in a UN uniform turns toward the camera as the word *witness* appears onscreen underneath his eyes. That's me.

Next came General Dallaire's turn. On the day of his interview he arrived in his Canadian Forces uniform with his tan-coloured UN uniform in a suit bag. The production team was assembled in a military reserve armoury just across the street from NDHQ. They had put up lights and camouflage nets in the drill hall to create the proper ambience. General Dallaire asked where he could change uniforms, so I brought him to the bathroom and held his suit bag while we chatted about the video. I knew that he was going through very rough times, and indeed he seemed a bit nervous about the interview. At one point he looked me right in the eyes and asked what I wanted him to say. I paused for a moment before telling him that if he wanted the video to have a real impact he had to say exactly how he felt: if he wasn't honest and transparent about his struggles with PTSD, then how could we ask front-line troops to ask for help? After a few minutes of discussion we agreed that it was necessary for him to be as candid as possible.

We went out to the drill hall and I stood back while Jamie conducted the interview. There, for the first time, a high-ranking Canadian officer admitted he had been in therapy for almost a year on account of the suicidal thoughts he'd had as a result of his time in Rwanda. General Dallaire, like many others, was facing an ongoing battle with the sights, sounds, and smells of that fateful tour. The entire scene was very poignant and powerful. The general displayed a new type of courage that day by putting his own career and reputation on the line to show others that it was okay to show vulnerability.

Because of the video's candid nature, a copy of the final script was sent to the office of the military's judge advocate general for review, to ensure that the soldiers' testimonies didn't cause any legal problems. Shortly after, it was sent back to me with a list of suggested changes to General Dallaire's words. I called and tried to explain that the only way to edit Dallaire's testimony was to reshoot the scene, which wasn't in the budget. The military's lawyers were quite concerned about a three-star general discussing suicidal thoughts on camera, and the argument was only put to rest when Dallaire himself weighed in and said he wanted it left alone.

Ultimately, *Witness the Evil* was one of the first shots fired at the wall of silence that guarded the subject of mental health in the Canadian military. The honesty displayed by Dallaire and other Canadian peacekeepers was a significant catalyst for the changes that followed over the next several years.

THROUGHOUT 1997 AND 1998 things moved at a quick pace. In spite of the fact that I was a psychological mess, I'd gone on several overseas tours, had completed work on *Witness the Evil*, and I was even up for promotion. But there were a few hiccups along the way that made me unpopular with some of my colleagues.

One occurred in the fall of 1997. In June of that year I, along with a team of seven other public affairs staff and a French editor, were cited for a commendation by the deputy minister of national defence. Our team had recently helped with a report to the prime minister by communicating the MLO's initiatives to the public and the Canadian Forces. Since the department was constantly trying to put a positive spin on anything it could, my superiors made a mountain out of a mole hill. We'd simply done our jobs, and yet here I was, a glorified bureaucrat, being recognized for pushing paper, when in my mind I'd done a lot more impactful work in Rwanda that few people cared about at all.

After giving it some thought, I informed my boss, a colonel, that I wouldn't be attending the ceremony. He was unhappy about my decision and he ordered me to attend, but I remained steadfast in my decision. And yet, in spite of my recalcitrance, I was promoted to major later that spring. With the promotion came a move to Toronto and a posting to Land Force Central Area Headquarters (LFCAHQ). So in the spring of 1998 Julie, the kids, and I packed up our home and moved to a little bungalow in the Toronto suburb of Etobicoke. When we arrived, our elderly Polish landlady told us that she only rented to military personnel; she knew if the rent went unpaid the military would take action against the offender. (She must've had some bad experiences with civilian tenants.) The house was very affordable and had a big backyard (a rarity in Toronto), so we were quite happy with the change. I also got to work with some great people at LFCAHQ. All in all, I felt things were looking up.

The problem, though, was that LFCAHQ existed mainly for domestic operations—natural disasters and the like; in peacetime things were pretty boring. I liked the people I worked with, but how could routine work be taken seriously after Rwanda, my NDHQ intrigues, and several other overseas tours? Life started to feel tedious.

WITHIN SIX MONTHS of starting my appointment I was showing signs of severe stress. Boredom at my job, living in a hectic city, and a lack of motivation gave my inner demons plenty of opportunity to surface and torture my mind. Once a week, in the morning, branch heads (which included me) met to discuss ongoing domestic operations, exercises, and policies with our chief of staff, Colonel Chris Corrigan. My daily route to work involved a bike ride to the Islington subway station and then a forty-five minute subway ride to Yonge Street and Finch Avenue. To make things easier I travelled in civilian clothing and then used the showering facilities at work to change into my uniform.

One morning I was on the subway, reading a book and waiting for the train to depart, when I had an eerie feeling that someone was watching me. I lowered my book, peered upward, and saw a black man sitting directly across from me, staring. I went back to my book, but as I tried to absorb the words part of me kept wondering, "What's he looking at?" When I glanced up again he was still looking at me. My brain suddenly went into a cycle of paranoid and irrational thoughts. The man began to look like the major who'd threatened me in my office near the end of my time in Rwanda. Indeed, I was convinced that the man on the subway recognized me—why else would he be staring at me? Maybe he was there to assassinate me, I thought. What if he knew where I lived? Then he could harm my family, too. A kaleidoscope of thoughts and emotions took over as I sat there, utterly confused and fearing for my life.

Suddenly, as if only a second had gone by, I was back to reality and standing on Yonge Street. At first I had no idea where I was or what I was doing: I was nowhere near my office, and I had no clue how much time had elapsed. I had somehow jumped from the subway car to Yonge Street with no recollection of what had occurred in the interim. When I got my bearings I realized I was just north of the Eaton Centre, in Toronto's south end—more than fifteen kilometres from my office. I looked at my watch and saw that almost thirty minutes had passed since I saw the man staring at me from across the subway car. Where had I gone? What had I done? The past half-hour had been a total blur, as if I'd travelled into the future. Nevertheless, although I felt completely disoriented, I was worried about missing my morning meeting, and so I rushed to the nearest station and rode to work for the second time. After all, I couldn't say to my boss, "Sorry, sir, I was avoiding a Rwandan assassin on the subway." In the end, by the time I arrived, showered, and changed, the meeting was almost finished.

An interesting thing happened in the wake of that episode. Colonel Corrigan pulled me aside after the meeting finished and asked me to stick around. Given my late arrival I assumed that I was in trouble. Instead, we went to his office and had a really great conversation. Having read my personnel file he told me, very tactfully, that the excellence reflected in it did not match the man sitting in front of him. He said that he was concerned, and that he understood Rwanda was a difficult tour. He then told me that he wanted to give me all the time I needed to take care of myself and address whatever issues were going on in my head. He concluded by saying that he was prepared to email the medical surgeon and ask if she could set up an appointment for me to speak with someone.

The colonel was my superior, but he'd acted more like a peer during our conversation. It was as if he'd given me the permission to start recovering from my turmoil. Up to then, the military rarely acknowledged that mental health issues even existed; the few times it did, sufferers were quickly swept under the rug to avoid any potential scandal. Indeed, those of us who had problems functioning were usually either ignored or shunned like lepers. Strictly speaking I didn't *need* permission to recover, but the colonel's support was a precipitating moment for me. Like my conversation with Alain Ouellette a few years earlier, Colonel Corrigan's skillful handling of my condition gave me a taste of the potency of peer support.

Ironically, when the medical surgeon contacted me, she offered to set up an appointment with the very psychiatrist I'd seen a few years earlier. I baulked at this suggestion, and in the end she provided me with an alternate choice: Dr. David Prendergast, a civilian psychologist whom I saw for almost a year. I didn't know it yet, but my road to recovery had finally begun in earnest.

IN THE FIRST few months after returning from Rwanda in March 1995 I dealt with nightmares and several other symptoms that, in the twenty-first century, would cause any medical professional to say, "That's classic PTSD." Yet by the time I began therapy with Dr. Prendergast, in the summer of 1999, my illness had evolved into something different. I certainly felt a tinge of survivor's guilt after witnessing so much death and destruction, but the bulk of my struggle had to do with a more general need for order. I was always the kind of person who wanted to be punctual and follow the rules, but as time went by I somehow lost my ability to keep things in perspective. To my mind, being one minute late to a meeting was now as bad as showing up an hour late at the airport and missing your flight. This inability to properly sort out the merely inconvenient from the devastating had been pulling me down like a lead weight.

Put simply, things were either great or gut-wrenching—there was no middle ground. I was undergoing treatment for PTSD, and I had already been dealing with depression, but I started to believe something else was going on, too, something not mentioned in the *Diagnostic and Statistical Manual of Mental Disorders*. Few of the clinicians I had spoken with thus far understood what was happening, and those that did tried to place it under the catch-all PTSD umbrella. Their treatment methods and understanding came close, but not close enough. I eventually came to believe it was time to rethink "trauma."

A NEW PATH opened up in my life as I began my healing journey with Dr. Prendergast. But I wasn't content with just figuring out what was wrong with *me*: I also wanted to fix the whole military mental health system. When I wasn't at my day job at LFCAHQ I spent almost all my free time conducting Internet searches and reading books. One day I came across the name of Dr. Arieh Shalev, one of the world's leading PTSD experts, whose research looks at psychological trauma in the Israeli Defense Forces. Dr. Shalev, who I soon learned was a kind and patient man, got more than he bargained for when he responded to my first email query, since a barrage of others soon followed. My goal was now to uncover everything there was to know about mental health, PTSD, and its antecedents like "shell shock." My new obsession coincided with an increasing awareness, since my return from Rwanda, of soldier suicides. By the late 1990s, several soldiers I'd served with had committed suicide; this weighed on my heart and also made me angry because it was so unnecessary. In combination with my own negative experiences with the military's health system, I decided that things needed to change.

One morning I arrived at work to find an incident report pertaining to a soldier's suicide. The man was a master corporal from the Royal Canadian Regiment. They found his body hanging from a tree in Algonquin Provincial Park. For some reason, that particular suicide really upset me, and so I rose from my desk and walked to the command cell, a secluded area of the building where General Walter

Holmes's office was. When I arrived there I bumped into the general's executive assistant, a major who was also from the Royal Canadian Regiment. He was a nice but traditional guy from the "suck it up" school of thought. I asked if he had heard the news, to which he casually replied, "Yeah." He didn't appear to be concerned, even when I said that it seemed like every month we were hearing about another suicide. I then asked if he knew the soldier in question. He turned to me, and without even a moment's thought denounced the man as a drunk and an idiot.

My anger began to grow. I asked pointedly whether the man who committed suicide was always a drunk, and how many tours he had completed before his death. The major said the man had definitely had good days, and he'd served on several tours, including one in Somalia and two in Bosnia. I looked him in the eye and with an impatient tone asked why he would denounce such a brave soldier as a mere drunk. His response was to laugh off my concern and dismiss the man's suicide as something that happened all the time. In his mind it was no big deal—just business as usual.

That conversation disturbed me almost as much as hearing about the suicide itself. How could an officer in the Canadian military, one from the *same regiment* as the man who killed himself, have absolutely no sympathy or empathy for one of his own? I went back to my office and sat there for almost an hour, pondering the major's indifference and what could be done to battle that sort of attitude. His casual, flippant response to such a serious subject reflected a broken system. In combination with my own battles with mental health, that discussion caused me to further intensify my research and to work toward some sort of lasting reform.

DR. PRENDERGAST SPECIALIZED in working with emergency medical workers, so he'd dealt with those who had first-hand experience with harrowing events. When I began seeing him in 1999 we talked often about things that happened in my daily life and what sorts of "triggers" exacerbated my illness—which sights, sounds, or smells sparked memories of traumatic events and/or aroused intense emotions. Dr. Prendergast was a very approachable therapist, and he did an excellent job of explaining to me how the brain processes information. Our discussions allowed me to begin wrapping my head around what "PTSD" really was. I still wasn't convinced that the concept captured the entirety of what I felt and experienced, but with an understanding of what triggers were and how they related to my brain's functioning, I was better able to cope when a sight or smell brought back unwanted memories of Rwanda.

I had a chance to see this in action on my drive home from work one afternoon in the fall of 1999. The day was unseasonably warm and I was on the highway with the windows down when I suddenly got a whiff of diesel fumes. It was as though I was smelling the diesel emanating from the old Land Rover I drove in Rwanda, and within seconds I'd been transported back to the country. But the smell of diesel suddenly morphed into the stench of dead bodies. For a few moments I was quite distressed. Undergoing such a frightful transformation on what was otherwise a regular drive home from work was unsettling, to say the least. But my treatment had given me the tools to bring myself back to reality, and as soon as I realized what was happening I used some of the grounding techniques Dr. Prendergast had taught me to refocus myself. Though rattled, I was now back on the highway in Toronto instead of stuck in the Rwandan countryside smelling bodies.

When I realized I had, for the first time, made it through a flashback without losing my cool, I felt like a kid who'd finally grasped that two plus two equals four. Some things seem so simple when you know them by heart, but when you are just learning them they can feel quite complex. I went home that night with a sense of comfort and pride: treatment was finally beginning to work. I was coping with intrusive memories, sights, and smells, and I was bringing meaning to what had happened in Rwanda by brainstorming changes to the military health system that would help others dealing with similar issues. In short, I had turned a corner and my new psychological prosthesis—my coping mechanisms and understanding of how to handle mental intrusions from Rwanda—was starting to fit well.

Chapter 5

FAMILY TROUBLES AND THOUGHTS OF SUICIDE

I t is necessary to pause for a brief interlude. While recounting my experience both during and after Rwanda, I've so far provided only brief glimpses of the depths to which my mind sank after 1995 and how these difficulties affected my family. It's now time that I open up about how I treated Julie and the kids as I battled suicidal thoughts after Rwanda. That battle lasted over ten years—and in fact, certain difficult memories from this period still occasionally flare up to this day.

After my return from Rwanda, on a beautiful, late-spring day in 1995, Julie went off to visit her parents while I stayed home and took care of the kids. Veronique had outgrown her crib, so I decided to use the day to make her a little princess bed. Since we lived on a dead-end street I didn't have to worry about traffic, so I let her wheel her tricycle around on the road while I worked in the garage with the door open. David, who was always curious about what his dad was doing, watched intently as I began my work. He soon became insistent about helping in some way, so I gave him his toy hammer and put a wooden two-by-four with a few nails on the ground for him to hit. As far as he

93

knew he was helping make the bed. Once Veronique looked over and saw her brother, it wasn't long before she decided that she, too, wanted to help.

I worked away for the next hour while the kids played in the garage, sometimes watching me, sometimes walking in and out, other times banging away on David's two-by-four. But as the minutes went by I grew more anxious about the noise and their presence. I was relatively handy at carpentry, and building furniture was not something I normally found difficult, but that day I was having a tough time concentrating: things just weren't coming to me the way they normally did. As the kids buzzed around me I cut a piece of wood, and then subsequently realized that it was too short, which only added to the frustration building up inside me. David was hammering again, and he became impatient because he wasn't able to drive the nail into the board. He started to cry, and I tried to comfort him as best I could, but inside me a kettle began to boil.

I don't remember exactly what finally set me off, but I recall glaring at David and thinking: "Holy shit, stop making so much noise!" When he looked back at me I could see for a brief moment that he understood my face had suddenly changed. I clawed my fingers into my head and yelled, "DAVID, STOP IT!" Both kids immediately ceased what they were doing, stared at me for a moment, and then broke down crying. I grabbed David by the shoulders and shook him, not very hard but enough to scare him. I repeated: "STOP IT, DAVID, JUST STOP IT!" This only freaked him out even more. Thankfully, after a few seconds I came to my senses.

In the end I'd scared him more than I'd hurt him, but it must've been terrifying for both him and Veronique nonetheless. I apologized and said that I didn't know what had happened, which was quite literally true. But even though I didn't know I was sick, I knew my reaction was out of character. I decided the best thing to do was stop building the bed, bring everything inside the garage, and go back into the house. The rest of the afternoon went well and I spent some time playing with the kids in the living room, but I was disturbed by my outburst. I never had a temper like that before my Rwanda tour. I knew enough to know that what I'd done wasn't a good thing, and I worried that the kids were going to grow up maladjusted if I continued having these types of episodes.

I had a similar incident with David years later, in 2003, when he was a teenager. We were living in Cantley, a rural municipality north of Gatineau that is only about twenty kilometres from Ottawa. One afternoon I decided to come home early, since things were slow at work. I usually made it home well after the kids were done school, but because I'd left early I arrived at the same time as David. As I pulled into the driveway his bus was right behind me. I took my briefcase out of the car, and we exchanged the usual greetings while walking up to the front door. David was pulling his usual rebel-without-a-cause, cool-guy routine, as many teenage boys do. When we got to the porch I went to unlock the door, and I heard the sound of him spitting his gum onto the ground.

I looked down at the gum on the front porch and became instantly overwhelmed. Julie and I were strict parents when the kids were young, always making sure they behaved in restaurants and respected others. David's small act of spitting his gum out became a trigger, one that aroused intense emotions within me. When I later spoke to my psychiatrist, Dr. Peter Boyles, he said that I took David's action as a defiance of my authority. Perhaps I did. But in the moment what overpowered me was a sense that somehow David's gesture would lead to complete chaos. There was no middle in my mind between behaving well and genocide. As soon as he crossed the line from good behaviour to bad there was potential for complete civil disobedience and breakdown. That mentality made no sense to a rational person, but the minute I saw someone disrespecting proper manners or customs, whether it was bullying in the workplace or not following "the rules," I lost it. In my mind, complete harmony and complete chaos were the only two states that existed.

My inner temperature immediately went to boiling, but I nonetheless calmly asked David what he was doing. Being a teenager, he replied nonchalantly by asking me what I meant. I explained that spitting gum on the porch was a ridiculous thing to do, and after a few excuses he apologized, then promptly picked it up and flung it onto the grass. Now I was even more impatient, though I still managed to keep my cool, at least on the outside. I told him to pick it up and put it in the garbage can inside. Hearing my tone, he reluctantly complied before coming into the house.

Instead of following him in, I asked him to tell Julie that I had to return to work because I forgot something. That was a complete lie, but I knew that I needed to get out of the situation before I lost it. I immediately got in my jeep and drove back to work, talking myself down the entire time. Quite simply, I had no coping fuel left. I worried that if David somehow challenged me again things might escalate. I went back to work for a few hours and found some things to do while I tried to calm down. Julie called after she got home and asked where I was, so I explained what had happened. She understood, but she pointed out to me that what David did was no big deal. She asked me to come home, but I said I couldn't because I might blow up on him if he did or said anything more. As always she was very supportive, and she told me to take the time I needed and that dinner would be waiting when I got back.

I arrived home again after dark, and when I finished eating Julie insisted that I talk with David. He knew he had pushed my buttons, and he felt bad about it. David is a great kid, and when I spoke with him in the living room he told me he was sorry, that he didn't know that spitting out his gum would make me so upset. Even as a teenager he knew there was something not right with his dad, and during our conversation I could see him trying to understand and empathize with me. What still makes me emotional when recalling that day is that I could nonetheless see guilt in his eyes, as if somehow the situation was in some way *his* fault. I tried to explain that I was messed up, and that I sometimes overreacted to things. Thankfully, we ended the conversation with a hug and there were no hard feelings. My coping had gotten a lot better than just after my return from Rwanda, but those situations still happened far more often than any father would want them to.

EVEN MORE WORRYING than my newfound temper and odd idiosyn-
crasies were the thoughts I'd developed about suicide. In the decade
after my return from Rwanda there were several occasions when I
came close to ending it all.

My first serious, sustained thoughts of suicide (as opposed to the
fleeting notion I'd had in the fall of 1995 about crashing my car) came
when I was alone one weekend in 2007. By this point David was off at
the University of Montreal; Veronique and Julie (who started teaching in 2004) were visiting family friends in Toronto. I was having a
good day amidst a stretch of really bad ones, but as the afternoon
went on I felt more and more weighed down, especially by the way my
fellow soldiers were being treated by the DND. Mental health issues
were being swept under the carpet, and in some cases, sufferers were
being released from the military without a pension. Coupled with my
personal struggles, my frustration at this situation made for a perfect
storm.

By the evening I felt something I had occasionally experienced
before, though never so intensely. I was lying on the couch listening
to music, but all I could think about were various ways to kill myself.
I obeyed a very measured and rational thought process as I went
through the strengths and weaknesses of each approach, and yet I
knew that something was terribly wrong. It was as if there were two of
me in the house—one lying on the couch contemplating suicide, and
another standing behind soundproof Plexiglas yelling at his alter ego
to snap out of it. The problem was, the two versions of me couldn't
understand each other.

After a few hours of lying there, a light bulb suddenly came on,
and I went online and searched under "ways to commit suicide." For
another hour I read several blogs and websites about suicide, each of
which contained tips about what methods to use: carbon monoxide
poisoning, prescription medications, and hanging are just some of
the most common. After weighing the pros and cons of each I thought
of something else. I had a few guns in the house; this seemed like the
most efficient, foolproof way. I got up, walked to the garage, and took
out my father's .303 rifle from the Second World War. I never actually

loaded it, but I put my mouth around the barrel and reached for the trigger, to figure out if it was possible to discharge the weapon from that angle. It was a bit of a stretch for my arm, which made me scared that I might not hit the right part of the brain, that I'd miss and end up paralyzed but still alive, or even worse, brain-damaged. I thought about pulling the trigger with a stick, but that didn't seem like a guarantee either.

After a lot of internal debate I realized that what I was doing wasn't good, and so I went back inside, where I wondered what to do about my suicidal thoughts. I looked up some resources online, but felt like I shouldn't bother the suicide hotline: in my mind, they probably had other people to help, and they would try to talk me down from the ledge, which in the moment wasn't what I wanted. Instead I walked back to the garage and began holding the rifle again. My impulses seemed to come and go like the wind. One minute I was ready to try suicide, the next I was back to my senses again. Thankfully, after playing with the rifle for a few more minutes the gravity of my thoughts hit me like a bolt of lightning. I thought to myself, "Oh my god, if I do this, what are Julie and Veronique going to find when they come home?"

Finally, I snapped out of it, put the rifle back, and shook my head as feelings of guilt and shame came over me. I spent the remainder of the night trying to recalibrate myself and rationalize what I'd done. Oddly, I felt no self-pity, no feelings of depression, not even a sense of urgency. The whole process had unfolded in a cold, deliberate, and rational way.

MY SECOND SUICIDAL episode occurred in the winter of 2009. Work was going well, and though Julie and I had drifted apart somewhat we still ran a very efficient household. The problem was, no matter how well life was going, I still encountered crescendos of intense mental fatigue. On the surface things were fine, but I was exhausted from constantly having to apply coping mechanisms. I could never just be myself—or at least my old self.

One evening after dinner I was puttering around the house while Julie marked French homework at the kitchen table. Wherever I went and whatever I did, I kept having thoughts of suicide. I felt like I couldn't deal with life anymore, like I would never find happiness or equilibrium again. As with my first episode, I felt no pity or despair—I simply felt like turning out the lights on life. I went to the garage and grabbed some paper that I normally used for creating wood projects, and I wrote out a suicide note, basically just a short message stating that I was done with it all. When I finished I went back inside the house and placed the note on a wine rack near the door. We didn't have papers lying around the house so I thought that would be a conspicuous place where Julie would see it.

I quietly exited the house, locked the door, got in the car, and drove off. My plan was to get on the highway, drive really fast, and hit a pillar. But when I started driving I had so many questions, just like when I'd thought about shooting myself: how fast would I have to drive to make sure the airbags wouldn't keep me alive? What angle should I hit the pillar at? After several minutes I got off the highway and drove around, trying to work out the details. But once again, as I debated things in my head, my better half was yelling from behind the Plexiglas for me to stop contemplating suicide and go home. I just couldn't understand him.

The Gatineau River was very close to our house; I thought that maybe I could just drive the jeep into the water and drown myself, but again I had doubts. Feeling aimless, I found a large parking lot and backed into a secluded space where I hoped to work out a plan. For half an hour I sat there with the car off. In the end, the lack of heat may have saved my life. Indeed, the cold seemed to bring me back into the moment (Canadian winters *are* good for some things, it turns out). When I started the jeep it dawned on me how foolishly I was acting. My sensible alter ego had finally broken through the Plexiglas.

Unfortunately, my relief was replaced by terror when I remembered that my suicide note was still on the wine rack. At that point it was almost 11:00 p.m., and all I could think about was how I needed to get home before Julie discovered the note. I raced home, and when

I arrived I saw the light on in the bathroom upstairs; this was a good sign, since it meant she'd probably gone straight upstairs without seeing the note. And sure enough, I breathed a deep sigh of relief when I saw the note still sitting where I'd left it. I grabbed it, rushed to the wood stove in the kitchen, and threw it in. With the evidence disposed of, I went upstairs and said hello to Julie. At that point in our relationship we weren't keeping close track of each other's activities. My struggles had driven a wedge between us, and in the years after my return from Rwanda it sometimes felt like we were strangers living under the same roof. So I didn't face any questions when I got into bed. She probably assumed I'd been at work. My secret was safe.

AFTER CONTINUING TO think about suicide for many days and nights I decided that hanging was probably the best method. It was summertime in Cantley, and sugar bush season was over. Like many people in rural Quebec, Julie and I had a sugar shack—a little shed where we boiled maple sap—in our backyard.* But aside from her throwing an annual spring party in it, I was the only one who ever used it. It was the perfect place. I could lock myself in and ensure that no one would stumble upon my body after I did the deed.

One Saturday afternoon I came up with a plan: I would write an email to the police on my cell phone, giving them my address and the details of where they could find me, and send it just before I hanged myself. I went to the garage, got a rope and a ladder, and brought it to the sugar shack. Julie was busy inside the house doing her usual weekend chores. She was accustomed to seeing me busy myself with home projects, and wouldn't have thought anything about seeing me carry a rope and ladder.

---

* Sugar shacks, also known as sugar houses, sugar cabins, sap houses, or *cabanes à sucres* in French, are common in rural parts of eastern Canada, especially Quebec. In the spring, sap is collected from sugar maple trees and boiled to make maple syrup. As with most families, we usually did our collection and production in April or May, to celebrate the fact that winter was over and that spring had begun.

Once I was in the shack I locked the door, positioned the ladder, and tied the rope to one of the large ceiling beams. I double checked the knots, and then came back down to look up the contact information for the local police. Once I found their email address I wrote a polite message saying that I had just committed suicide, and I concluded by apologizing for putting them through such a traumatic event. This might sound strange to those who've never had suicidal thoughts, but as I double-checked my preparations a feeling of complete contentedness came over me. I felt relieved that soon I wouldn't have to cope with the thoughts that had plagued me for years—the little girl with her head chopped into pieces, the little boy who'd been shot, the piles of bodies, and the confusion that so often accompanied these visions.

Many people misunderstand PTSD. They think that when a trigger occurs the person freaks out, and that when there are no triggers the person is fine. My experience was very different. For me, triggers were easy to deal with once I knew how. It was, rather, the exhaustion of trying to pretend I was okay that got to me. I felt an intense weight pushing down on me, and I could no longer remember what the point of life was. Unsurprisingly, I was also riddled with guilt over the genocide in Rwanda, and what, if anything, we could've done differently. Words fail me when I try to describe these feelings, but somehow I felt like my reality was not the same as everyone else's. I could try my best to be a good husband, father, and friend, but I could never truly enjoy life, even though I knew I should. That feeling became my norm. Most days I held it together because I knew I needed to for Julie and the kids, but over time it became more and more difficult to maintain the facade.

After a final check of my email to the police I was about to proceed when I heard a noise outside—footsteps in the gravel leading to the shack. As the steps got progressively louder I heard Julie calling my name. She sounded nervous. Maybe she was worried because the doors were closed: somehow, she always had a sixth sense for when things weren't right. Sure enough, she peered in through the window, saw the ladder and rope, and panicked. She started yelling frantically as she cupped her hands over her face and looked inside. I froze as her gaze met mine, like a kid who'd been caught red-handed doing something he wasn't supposed to. Right away my thoughts of suicide were replaced with intense guilt: "What have I done? I just really hurt my wife." Unfortunately, sometimes when you're suicidal one of the last things on your mind is how your actions will impact others. I never even thought about what would happen if she caught me before I went through with it.

I quickly opened the door and tried to comfort Julie, who was trembling. She wasn't sure what to do, and she asked if she should call the police or a suicide hotline. I told her everything was fine, and then I started to cry. She cried, too, and together we walked up to the house. Once inside I sat on the front hall stairs while she paced back and forth, repeatedly asking what she should do. I tried again to console her by telling her that the thought was gone, but this was a lie: the thought was never entirely gone, it just retreated from time to time to the edge of my consciousness. Despite my profuse apologies, I could still see despair in her face. Although we'd drifted apart we still loved one another, and I knew she felt guilty about not supporting me enough, even though she did absolutely everything she could, and more. That event had a huge impact on her, and I wish I could take it all back. Of course, I can't.

I'D LIKE NOW to briefly turn the microphone over to Julie. While preparing this book I felt it was important to have her input, and to give her the chance to relate these events in her own words. What follows is some of what she said about our life together after I returned from Rwanda in 1995, and how my illness affected her.

Although I didn't realize how much I'd changed as a result of my time in Rwanda, Julie noticed almost instantly. She saw that I was no longer the gregarious man I once was.

He became a loner, whereas he wasn't really before. And all outings pretty much stopped. He didn't mind people coming over, but I started to understand that it was because he could control the situation. What he did was retreat—retreat into himself. He didn't have much patience for other people. It was very instinctual. Basic survival, primal survival patterns. Oh, and then the home projects. All of a sudden he was knocking down walls and fixing things. There was so much activity—too much, in fact. And then, not long after he came back, he started volunteering for every mission that came about.

My odd and unpredictable behaviour took a heavy toll on Julie's life.

What happens to the spouse is that you become the protector of the one who's just trying to survive. But at the same time you know their behaviour is coming from a primal place. Their troubles are not shared with their family. So you become their connection to the outside world, their connection to their family, to their children, to their parents, and you start protecting them. You say things to the kids like, "Now we need to let him be," or "We need to respect his time alone."

Things got inexorably worse for her.

Eventually your world gets so small that there are no more outings. Our home life was like living in a cocoon for a long time. You become a caregiver to a young man, because he is a sick person. You care for the children and you care for your sick spouse. I took on all the roles inside the house, because he came up with a thousand projects to stay busy. I also took on more of the psychological aspects of taking care of things.

Julie persevered through many years of being the rock for our family, and it gradually wore on her.

I think, like most wives, you don't question it. You just say, "Well you gotta do what you gotta do." You make everything about everyone else, and then you forget yourself completely. You don't realize how much you've lost until much later in life, when the kids move out and you think, "What's left?" You suddenly realize, "Wow, I've completely forgotten myself here, and I don't know how to do anything else but *that*." Your caregiver role defines you, it defines your happiness. Most people in this situation don't talk to anybody, because few people understand when things look normal on the outside, and you don't want to burden anyone else with your problems. It becomes exhausting. You suffer yourself, and when the realization comes it's devastating. In my case it came with depression, weight loss, and confusion. I asked myself, "Okay, what's my role in life now? What do I do?" I felt a huge sense of loss. Eventually you stop and think, "I need someone to take care of *me* now."

I think that just like Stéphane will live with this for the rest of his life, so will I. It's impacted us both *so* much. It's just part of who I am and I'll live with that for the rest of my life. I think back on all the time that was spent living in not-so-harmonious periods, or alone. There was a lot of being alone—alone not just because your spouse is often physically gone, but alone because Stéphane retreated completely into himself. You are completely and utterly alone. I still carry that deep loneliness.

But despite these difficult struggles, Julie has tried to use the experiences and pain she felt to make positive changes for others.

I've learned a lot. And now I can communicate, I can talk about mental health and see other people with problems and not judge them right away. I can now say, "Okay, maybe something else is going on with them." That helps immensely. In my job as a school teacher I can now identify potential mental health problems in my classroom, and provide any sort of help I can to children who need it. The feeling of helping someone else going through what you went through is very fulfilling.

Education is crucial because once you understand and somewhat normalize mental health problems, they're not so scary anymore. We need to allow people to come together and talk about this. Had Stéphane and I been educated, provided with some kind of support right away, told what to expect, and been given the proper coping skills, and if I had known that every once in a while I needed to take time for myself, we all would've been much better off.

Although I will always feel pained by how much my illness, and my resulting actions, affected my family, I take some small comfort from hearing Julie put a positive spin on her experiences. "The aim," she says, "is to turn all the resentment and anger and disappointment into something positive, to change those feelings so they don't drag you down for the rest of your life. You can grow from the experience."

Well said, Julie.

Chapter 6

TIME FOR CHANGE

My story now shifts back to the late 1990s, and the appointments I had in Toronto with my psychologist, Dr. Prendergast. As I mentioned earlier, Dr. Prendergast was an insightful and effective therapist, and from our appointments I began to understand some of what was going on in my mind. He taught me a lot about mental injuries, and his passion for the subject was contagious. Over time, the interest I'd developed while making *Witness the Evil* in 1998 slowly became an obsession. I wanted to find out everything there was to know about PTSD, and what doctors and other health professionals were doing correctly and incorrectly. I also started to examine how the military, and later civilian organizations, could provide non-clinical care for those enduring mental injuries. I didn't want others to struggle as I did, and I didn't want people to have to suffer alone for a long time before seeking help. To this end I spent much of my spare time between 1998 and 2001 building what became known as the Operational Stress Injury Social Support program (OSISS).

In the reading I was doing on trauma and mental health I kept bumping into the concept of social support. Many studies I read about PTSD, the military, war, and reintegration ended with a statement on the need for social support, but they rarely went into much detail. I noticed that there was a gap here, and I wanted to dig deeper. Informal peer support had been very helpful to me on a few occasions; I knew it could be even more helpful if it was described, organized, and properly harnessed.

At roughly the same time Chris Brewin, a psychologist in London, England, concluded that a lack of social support was a significant risk factor in the development of PTSD. In 2000, Dr. Brewin, along with several co-authors, published a meta-analysis—an analysis of multiple studies to determine common conclusions/problems among them—of risk factors for PTSD. This came in handy as I started developing OSISS.

While living in Toronto and reading about trauma and mental health I travelled to Ottawa a few times, where I reconnected with two guys I'd kept in touch with from Rwanda, Warrant Officer Mike Williams and Sergeant Rick Noseworthy. Both were now based at Canadian Forces Base Petawawa, and both were in therapy. Williams, in particular, was quite unwell. After one of their therapy sessions at the National Defence Medical Centre in Ottawa, I took them out for lunch.

During our two-hour discussion I ran the peer support concept by them and pitched an idea about training veterans who'd been through hard times to help others. Mike and Rick were highly supportive of the idea, and they reiterated how difficult it was to relate to their families and doctors, how stigma prevented them from sharing their difficulties with anyone. Our meeting was a key moment for me, since I always felt that both men were extremely competent soldiers and individuals who'd been badly injured by stress: if they could be pushed to the brink, I reasoned, anyone could. Their enthusiasm inspired me to push on with my project to create a program for psychologically injured soldiers.

But why "Operational Stress Injury Social Support"? After beginning the project I flew to Halifax to attend a conference on PTSD, my goal being to figure out how I could stitch together a peer support program from the various research threads floating around the academic, corporate, and clinical worlds. At the conference I learned about a few corporate initiatives pertaining to peer support, which further piqued my interest about what current forms existed in Canada. Later, during a meeting with social worker Leah Greenwood, I also learned about the Gatehouse program, a peer support initiative launched in Toronto in 1998 that focused on helping survivors of childhood sexual abuse.

After examining numerous programs, I felt that two things were lacking. First, many were not flexible enough with their definition of "peer." In most cases, it simply meant co-worker. There was also a lot of talk about the Employee Assistance Program (EAP), and "peer referral" or "peer referral agents." Those "peers" were usually just trained in what the EAP could and couldn't do for co-workers. (Essentially, they were there to refer people to the EAP.) But they weren't concerned with having a non-clinical conversation with someone about their troubles, or supporting them on their path to recovery. In my estimation, peer support at the DND and within the military needed to be based on a program that utilized peers who'd been through the same ordeal as those they supported, similar to how cancer support groups were often led by cancer patients/survivors.

The second shortfall of most of these initiatives was the programmatic way they matched peer supporters with those needing help. For example, some programs required applicants to sign documents, which I knew wouldn't fly in a military setting, since soldiers were paranoid (rightfully so at the time) about anything that could end up on their service record or become public knowledge. Ultimately, while these existing models were nonetheless informative, providing me with much food for thought, they did not entirely fit with what injured veterans needed. A hybrid model was what these soldiers required, and this is what I hoped to create.

FOR OUR OFFICIAL unveiling of *Witness the Evil*, in 1998, the DND's public affairs department organized a cocktail party in Ottawa for participants and dignitaries. General Dallaire, who by this point was on sick leave for PTSD, could not attend the event, so Major-General Christian Couture attended in his stead. This was my first time meeting General Couture, and he immediately struck me as an approachable and likeable guy. He was a shorter man, a bit on the heavy side, and certainly did not project a traditional, tough-guy aura; but he nonetheless emanated a sense of competence, decisiveness, and caring leadership.

General Couture congratulated me on the release of the video, which he said was an important catalyst for change. This was somewhat surprising coming from a general, since at the time it seemed many of the military's high-ranking officers either denied that PTSD existed or tried to look the other way. Over the next few minutes I shared with him my concern about the social and medical challenges faced by soldiers with mental health issues. I hadn't yet learned concepts like "barriers to care" and other mental health lingo, but I was still able to express, in layman's terms, some ideas about how the military might address these challenges.

General Couture was very receptive about what I had to say. He had a hundred people to shake hands with that night, but he never once seemed to look across the room for a reason to break off our chat. I could tell he was genuinely intrigued. When the conversation finished he told me that he wanted to know more, and he invited me to expand on my ideas in a future meeting. I'd become obsessed with mental health, and my passion was fueled even more when I piqued the interest of a general who could help enact change from the top down. I returned to Toronto fired up, and I kept reading all I could about trauma, military culture, and programs for people with mental health issues. As it turned out, I would need the general's help in the coming days.

IN MARCH 2001, as I was continuing my research, Corporal Christian McEachern, a member of the Princess Patricia's Canadian Light Infantry who was suffering from PTSD, drove his sport utility vehicle through the doors of garrison headquarters at CFB Edmonton. Like many of his colleagues, Christian had had a rough time on overseas peacekeeping missions, and his experiences haunted him long after his return.* He was ostracized from his unit after developing psychological difficulties, and eventually, without any support from his peers or the institution, he had a mental breakdown. Driving his Nissan Xterra into a military office was the desperate act of a man who'd been abandoned by the organization he had given so much of his life and health to. From 2001 until the end of his trial in 2003, his story became a *cause célèbre* in national newspapers, one that shone a spotlight on the treatment of soldiers with mental injuries.

Throughout my own ordeal with stress and trauma, I always wondered what it would be like to deal with the same issues as a corporal or a private. As an officer, I enjoyed more latitude than those at the bottom of the military food chain. I certainly had trouble coping like anyone else, but because I had a lot more autonomy and flexibility, I could walk away for a few moments and take a breather during a really stressful day. Officers weave in and out of a heavily structured daily routine, one characterized by physical exercise, equipment maintenance, and many other mundane tasks. Non-commissioned members—that is, privates, corporals, and warrant officers—don't have that option. I couldn't help but wonder, how did people like McEachern get by?

In the days immediately after McEachern's story became national news, it occurred to me that his case presented a perfect opportunity for me to talk with someone who knew what it was like to suffer from PTSD as a non-commissioned member. I spoke to my boss in Toronto, Chris Corrigan, and, to my surprise, within a few days I was given permission to fly to Alberta and talk with McEachern in person. McEachern was posted to Land Force Western Area (comprised of the provinces of Manitoba, Saskatchewan, Alberta, and British Columbia); since this was a different chain of command from where I was posted in Toronto, my "mission" was very unorthodox by military standards. It wasn't every day that an officer from the central area of

---

*   For those interested in learning more about McEachern's story, both the *National Post* and the *Globe and Mail* provided coverage throughout the 2001–03 period.

Canada flew west to discuss mental health with a non-commissioned member in Alberta, and I'm sure some people wondered why I was doing this. Whatever the reason, my request was approved; it was a fortuitous and welcome development.

When my flight landed in Edmonton I discovered that Chris wasn't at home, but rather at the Alberta Hospital, a large psychiatric hospital in the northeastern part of the city. So I rented a car at the airport and drove straight there to visit him, using the trip to contemplate what I should say when I arrived. Despite having seen psychiatrists and psychologists in an office setting, I'd never seen a psychiatric hospital except in the movies, and I didn't know what to expect. Upon arrival I showed the hospital staff my military ID, explained why I was there, and was floored when a nurse commented, "Well, it's about time." Incidentally, Chris had been transferred to the Alberta Hospital after spending a few days in jail, and since then no one from the military had visited. I was embarrassed and ashamed, not just because my uniform represented the organization that had treated him so poorly, but also because as a human being I could only imagine the fear and loneliness that must have pervaded his mind as he sat alone in a psychiatric hospital, contemplating his fate.

The nurse wrote my name down and then quickly disappeared into the closed ward. She returned a few minutes later, said Christian would see me, and asked if I wanted to take him out for the day. I eagerly signed my name, essentially taking responsibility for ensuring he returned later that day. I was very nervous while I waited for him. Would he be embarrassed? Would he see me as part of the system and just tell me off? I was dressed in civilian clothing so as not to project an official look, but I didn't know if that would make any difference. I had no way of knowing whether he would even give me the time of day, and if my entire visit had been in vain.

Chris came out a minute later. He was polite as he shook my hand, but I could tell from his expression that he was wondering what the hell I was doing there; the fact that I was wearing jeans and a T-shirt instead of my military uniform must have added to his bewilderment. We chatted for a few minutes, and I told him that my main reason for visiting was to spend the day with him and pick his brain about what it was like to have PTSD as a non-commissioned member of the military. I described the peer support organization I envisioned, and I said that any input he could provide would be appreciated.

When I asked what he most wanted to do with his day out, he replied without hesitation that he wanted to see his dog. We had until 5:00 p.m., so we agreed to go get his dog, have lunch, and spend the afternoon discussing his predicament. We went to a local dog park, and while his dog played around we talked about the lead-up to Chris's incident at CFB Edmonton.

Later, over lunch, we discussed the possibility of a program for soldiers dealing with mental injuries. Chris spoke of the need he had to be connected with others who understood his feelings. Like many of his comrades with mental health problems, he'd thought that he was the only one on the planet who felt the way he did.

Throughout our conversation I could see that my ideas really spoke to Chris. I had discussed the program's development with numerous people by that point, but hearing the opinions of someone who'd been through the wringer as badly as Chris had was a landmark moment for me. I left our meeting more inspired about what a peer support program could offer soldiers in need, and I hoped that one day no one else would have to go through what Chris and numerous other comrades had experienced. As far as I was concerned, McEachern's case was the straw that broke the camel's back, the signal that things *had to change*. To this end, on my flight back to Toronto the next day I drafted an email to General Couture outlining my ideas for him again and asking for his support.

But I should offer a brief addendum to the McEachern meeting. I was appalled to learn a few years later that the psychiatrist whom I first saw after returning from Rwanda had agreed to fly to Alberta to testify for the Crown against McEachern, despite having never even met him. By that point—this was in 2002–03—OSISS was well established, and I'd taken on a de facto advocacy role for mentally injured soldiers. I tried, unsuccessfully, to put a stop to the psychiatrist's actions: you don't send a high-ranking military psychiatrist to testify against one of your own; what kind of message does that send to soldiers with PTSD or other mental health issues?

At the trial, the psychiatrist testified that McEachern was well aware of his actions on the night he drove his SUV into the garrison, and that he'd simply acted in a drunken rage. The defence, supported by McEachern's psychiatrist, retired lieutenant-commander Greg Passey, countered that McEachern was in a PTSD-related dissociative state, something that could be proven by his having spent a few hours after his arrest curled up in a fetal position under the bed in his jail cell. Ultimately, McEachern was found guilty, but that didn't change the fact that several psychiatrists told me that unless they were subpoenaed they would never willfully testify against a current or former Canadian Forces patient, because such an action undermined any confidence patients and *potential* patients had in the military's medical system. So much for the patient's best interests. This only reaffirmed my earlier decision to break off treatment. I later read an article by Calgary attorney Benjamin Kormos that examined the McEachern case. Kormos took the psychiatrist to task for testifying against McEachern despite having a very limited knowledge of the case or McEachern's medical history.

A WEEK AFTER I sent my email to General Couture he replied and told me to book some meeting time with him during my next visit to Ottawa. But I couldn't wait. I immediately went to Chris Corrigan and asked if I could travel to Ottawa and pitch my idea to the general. He was a supportive boss, and he approved my trip on the spot. I then booked a half-hour meeting with General Couture before flying to Ottawa. Being a general, he was a very busy man, with people knocking at his door every ten or fifteen minutes for signatures, approvals, and other business pertaining to those high in the chain of command.

When I arrived at his office there were several other people scheduled for meetings, so I was unsure about whether there would be enough time to get out everything I wanted to say. I fidgeted nervously in the waiting area, but after a few minutes my name was called. After some initial pleasantries, I was surprised when the general asked me how Chris Cassavoy was doing. Chris, as you'll recall, was my driver in Rwanda; he was also a participant in *Witness the Evil*, and he'd spoken briefly with the general during the release party. How did the general remember a short chat with a corporal that happened a few years ago? He must've met hundreds or thousands of people in that time. This was surely a testament to the general's concern for the men and women under his command.

He remained very engaged as I explained my ideas for a peer support program, and he was even patient when confronted with the meandering nature of my thoughts. Indeed, when my thirty minutes were up, and his secretary knocked to tell him that his next meeting was waiting, he calmly looked up and said, "We're not done here."

In the end, the meeting lasted several hours—so long, in fact, that around noon he pulled out his lunch and ate while I continued my pitch. At one point he ran out of note paper and used one of his napkins (complete with mustard stains) to draw a line with an arrow and several dots along it. "So let me get this straight," he said. "When a soldier is physically injured, there is a quick intervention [dot], treatment [dot], and movement to this point [the end of the arrow]?" Then he drew another line below, this time with a lot of space between the dots: "What you're telling me is that when a soldier has a significant psychological problem, it could be years between the time when it occurs and when he recognizes he needs help?" "Exactly," I replied. He looked at me for a few seconds, and then matter-of-factly stated, "That's just not right."

We continued discussing the issue, and he expressed hope that the program I was proposing could shrink the amount of time between soldiers' first troubles and their recognition of needing help. We also agreed that the ultimate strategic goal was to align the way the military treated *mental* injuries with the way it treated *physical* injuries. Unless both were handled in a similar manner, those with mental health problems would never be granted the same chance to recover as those with a broken leg or a bad back. Peers who'd experienced mental health challenges and were on a path to recovery could help facilitate that objective.

When the meeting concluded, General Couture expressed enthusiasm for the program, and he also made several executive decisions on the spot, which included posting me from my current unit to the Canadian Forces College (also in Toronto) so that I could dedicate myself full-time to the project. Of course, I promptly accepted. That decision allowed me to avoid any distractions from my current job. I was elated. After many months of reading, researching, and brainstorming, I had finally been given a green light from someone in a leadership role.

When I walked out of the general's office the people waiting to see him were all looking at me, wondering what had taken so long and whether I was some kind of VIP. As a young major, the whole thing was somewhat surreal: a two-star general had just given me three hours of his time and approved a sharp turn in my career path on the spot. Another officer could just as easily have dismissed my idea, or simply said, "I don't really care about mental health, that's what doctors are for." But General Couture instinctively understood that the whole subject was connected to effective leadership. He knew that we needed to build relationships with doctors and other health specialists within the Canadian Forces, and that, at the end of the day, we needed a program with a non-clinical component and support from high-ranking officers—soldiers just wouldn't subscribe to it otherwise.

From then on, I thought of mental health in the workplace as a leadership issue. Clinicians were there to treat people when they were sick or having emergencies, but keeping them healthy *in the workplace*, and transforming the culture so that there were no barriers to care, was the responsibility of organizational leaders. We live in a democratic society, but most of our institutions are still structured so that the ability to make decisive changes often rests solely with those at the top. One inspired leader who is willing to cast off old ideas and bureaucratic inertia can therefore make a big difference in the lives of his or her employees.

I couldn't help but see my meeting with General Couture as a fateful moment in my life. Within a few weeks his decisions had been implemented, and I was on my way to officially forming the new peer support program.

ONCE I WAS posted to the Canadian Forces College I began working from home, dedicating myself full-time to the creation of a new organization for psychologically injured soldiers. My posting to the college was simply to give me the status I needed within the Canadian Forces to develop the program; I was actually accountable to the director of the Casualty Support Administration in Ottawa, Lieutenant-Colonel David Wrather. Thankfully, I discovered early on that Dave was very supportive of what I was doing. I now had the mandate to make sure the organization I'd envisioned was truly effective for those with mental injuries. Overall, I felt like things were finally coming together.

After I started my new posting at the Canadian Forces College in the summer of 2001, I happened to be in Ottawa on business when I ran into General Couture in the hallways of NDHQ. When he asked me how my project was going I responded by comparing my situation to the dog you always see chasing the school bus as it picks kids up for school: put simply, I'd caught the bus, but I didn't know what to do with it. This was my subtle way of telling him, "Holy shit, this project is intimidating." He laughed and patted me on the back. "One day at a time, Stéphane. One day at a time."

As I shaped the program, the relatively new Canadian Forces ombudsman's office (created in 1998) was investigating how the military treated soldiers with PTSD. It had become clear over the past several years, especially after peacekeeping missions during the 1990s, that the military's treatment of soldiers with PTSD was woefully outdated. One of the advisors on the investigation was retired brigadier-general Joe Sharpe, who'd been chairman of a military board of inquiry into whether Canadian soldiers had been exposed to toxins in Croatia in the mid-1990s. The board, which completed its investigation in January 2000, concluded that overwhelming levels of stress, and not toxins, were the likely culprit behind many soldiers' health issues. When Sharpe and the ombudsman's lead investigator, Gareth Jones, heard about my project, they contacted me for a meeting. For many in the military, the ombudsman's office was the anti-Christ, since it shone a spotlight on military culture and the inner workings of the chain of command, but I was unhappy with how mentally injured soldiers were being treated, so I saw the ombudsman's investigations as a step in the right direction.

When I met with Sharpe and Jones we immediately hit it off. Nevertheless, I couldn't help recall the fact that the ombudsman's report into the McEachern case indirectly took credit for having pushed the DND to create the peer support program. That always left me a little miffed, because it was entirely untrue. General Couture had not read the ombudsman's report—indeed, it had not even been produced yet when he decided to create what became OSISS. Uninformed people reading the report probably concluded, "Well, thank God the ombudsman did that report, because otherwise the DND never would've created the OSISS program." I beg to differ.

As I worked on what would become OSISS, Sharpe and Gareth, who were interviewing numerous members of the military suffering from PTSD, connected me with soldiers who they felt could provide some insights into what needed to change. One was Jean-François Laroche, an infantry warrant officer in the Royal Twenty-second Regiment, based out of Valcartier, Quebec. We spoke on many occasions, and it quickly became clear that he was really unwell and very isolated. As with many comrades during the 1990s, Jean-François had been involved in several harrowing operations, including Bosnia, Haiti, East Timor, and he'd been involved in front-line service during the 1990 Oka Crisis. He was a hero and an exemplary leader who'd become persona non grata when the military turned on him for developing PTSD. Since I was working out of Toronto and he was in Quebec, I provided what was essentially peer support over the phone every two weeks or so, and even more often than that when he was in crisis.

One day in the winter of 2001 I went to pick up some OSISS business cards at a printing shop when I was informed that the batch had been misprinted; instead of having all of the program's information, the cards were blank save for the OSISS logo. The shop's employee apologized and offered to throw them away, but I said I'd find a use for them somehow. A week later I had a long phone conversation with Jean-François, who was feeling very discouraged and isolated. I hung up the phone not knowing if I'd said the right things or been helpful— never a good feeling when dealing with those who are upset. I decided that perhaps it was best to make some kind of tangible gesture, so that Jean-François could *visibly* see that he had support. I reached in my desk and took out one of the blank business cards. In French I wrote: "To Jean-François: You are not alone! Call me anytime, Stéph."

I put the card in an express courier envelope, shipped it to his home, and soon forgot about it. Three years later I was at Ste. Anne's Hospital in Quebec, where Jean-François was going through treatment with other veterans.* He told me that earlier in the week he went to a group therapy session at which he'd been asked what had helped the most when he was at his lowest point: Jean-François calmly reached into his wallet and pulled out the business card I'd sent him, and which he'd kept with him ever since. I was greatly touched by his story. During OSISS's formative years I still didn't have a firm grasp on what peer support entailed. Sending the business card was the only tangible thing I felt that I could do, but I had no idea how meaningful and symbolic it would be to him. This anecdote taught me that one small conversation or gesture can make all the difference when someone is in despair.

When the OSISS program first launched we started with three initial sites—Petawawa, Winnipeg, and Edmonton. I also began to recruit my first peer supporters. With time, formal standards for the selection of peer supporters were established, but in the early stages of the program I picked them the old fashioned way—using gut instinct.

---

* Ste. Anne's has served Canadian veterans since it was founded in 1917, during the First World War.

My choice for the Petawawa site was Rick Noseworthy. I knew Rick from our Rwanda days, and he had all the qualities and experience that the position required. My choice for the Winnipeg site was Mike Spellen, an outstanding peer supporter recommended to me by Joe Sharpe. Mike, who served on the military's inquiry into Canadian peacekeepers' experiences in Croatia, had witnessed firsthand what harrowing moments did to soldiers when he served as a peacekeeper in the Balkans. He had worked closely with General Sharpe, and the two had become good friends. For the Edmonton site the chain of command immediately referred me to Corporal Greg Prodaniuk. Greg was a very polite, diplomatic advocate for people suffering from PTSD, and the chain of command felt he had the skills and competency for the job. I concurred.

Initially I chose to launch OSISS as a unilingual program, not because I didn't care about francophones (I am one after all!), but because there was so much to do, and I didn't know how to make the program bilingual right off the bat. Once the first peer supporters were chosen, and I had our budget and finances in order, I consulted again with the Toronto social worker Leah Greenwood on how to develop the program's training. Accountability was essential, since some in the military were watching like hawks for any missteps that they could use as an excuse to decrease funding or close the program down. To this end, training was scheduled for February 2001; the pilot program would commence a few months later.

One evening in the winter of 2001 I returned from a trip to Ottawa to find a voicemail from a soldier named Sean Hearn, who lived in Newfoundland. Julie, who first heard the message, said I should talk to him; judging from his voicemail, she thought he had something to offer the program. Although Julie was not officially involved, she followed the progress of my work carefully, so her thoughts meant a lot to me. I called Sean the next day, and after a half-hour conversation he convinced me that we should not launch the pilot program without at least a part-time peer supporter in Newfoundland and Labrador. He was the natural fit for that position.

The peer supporter course was set up during the summer and fall of 2000, and in February 2001 we had a two-week course led by Leah Greenwood. One key player during that time was Kathy Darte from Veterans Affairs Canada, who saw the value in partnering with us and extending peer support services to veterans as well as current soldiers. She became essentially my co-manager. Another important figure was retired lieutenant-colonel Jim Jamieson, a former military social worker who was very enthusiastic about new approaches to stress injuries. In 1997 Jim had produced a report on the care of injured soldiers and their families for the DND, and he was one of the first to recognize that the current system was flawed and outdated.

Jim, Kathy, and I became a team. We slowly stitched together a policy piece that outlined what OSISS strove for, how it would achieve its mission, and what it brought to the table—namely, a new approach to mental health and support for psychologically injured soldiers. This was meant to bring some accountability to our endeavour, and to explain what the program was all about. We knew that things would evolve over time, but we still felt it was better to have eighty per cent of something rather than a hundred per cent of nothing, so we launched with a few basic rules, regulations, and role descriptions for everyone to abide by.

BEFORE OSISS'S CREATION the term *operational stress injury* did not exist. When I began researching psychological trauma and mental "disorders," the military's refusal to accept that the mind could be prone to injury seemed quite strange. What I discovered was that the problem wasn't related to medical thinking, but rather to the military's organizational culture. The biggest contributor to the military's reticence to accept mental disorders was the word *disorder* itself. Every soldier I spoke with about the subject said that being told they had a disorder was devastating. And why wouldn't it be? After all, armies are largely about order—order pervades the entire organization in one way or another. Using the term *disorder* in such a culture is completely inappropriate and unnecessarily stigmatizing towards those who believe that order—and all that it entails—is such an important concept. Telling a soldier that he or she has a disorder is akin to telling them they are out of order. To add to the problem, unless those who know the soldier with the disorder happen to be a psychiatrist or psychologist, the term makes them feel completely powerless to help. Disorder is a medical term for medical professionals to utilize, and it does little good in military culture.

For these reasons I felt that the military needed a non-medical term that soldiers could understand and associate with their condition, something that didn't smack of doctors' jargon and "disorderly" behaviour. While reading a book by Dr. Allan English, a former Royal Canadian Air Force navigator and a historian at Queen's University— it covered the history of flying stress in Canadian aircrews during the Second World War—I was struck by how the word *injury* came up on several occasions. As I continued I started to believe that this word was far better for promoting a greater acceptance of the problems of the mind. Soldiers are used to dealing with injuries; after all, everyone has been injured at some point in their life, and in a physically demanding culture like the military an injury doesn't automatically carry a stigma.* Moreover, when soldiers and civilians encounter an injured person, they (usually) actively attempt to help the person in any way they can. I therefore felt strongly that if we rebranded "disorders" as "injuries" we could start the slow but deliberate process of shifting military culture from one of abdication to one of support.

Lastly, the new term needed to be generic enough to include injuries suffered during *any* operation, whether they were wars or peacekeeping missions. Prior to the late 1990s, most people felt that peacekeeping missions could not be injurious to the mind—indeed, some still believe this. Until the end of the Cold War, peacekeeping was generally viewed as an easy task. Only those who went to an official war were deemed worthy of developing psychological difficulties. But

---

*   Though of course in the military's hyper-masculine culture, even physical injuries are sometimes treated as something worthy of the phrase "suck it up buttercup."

after missions like those in the former Yugoslavia and Rwanda, the military chain of command, along with the Canadian public, gradually began to recognize that peacekeeping could be as stressful as war. We needed to reflect that development, and the word *operational* seemed to bring all types of missions under the same umbrella.

After much deliberation I therefore decided on "operational stress injury"; and given my conviction that social support was often the missing link for those with mental difficulties, I decided to add "social support" to the program's name as well. Thus, the term *operational stress injury* (OSI) was created and the Operational Stress Injury Social Support program was born. The latter name was a bit of a tongue twister, but the program was on its way, and "operational stress injury" stuck. Of course, some clinicians were offended that I'd made up a term, that since I had neither a doctorate nor a medical degree I'd overstepped my role as a soldier. The concept of operational stress injuries, and my competency, were challenged on many occasions by those who believed that I was trampling on sacred medical ground. On those occasions, perhaps with a bit of arrogance, I told them off, explaining that the term was not a clinical concept, but was for us— the members of the military. And yet, to my surprise, Veterans Affairs later decided to apply the OSI designation to their mental health clinics. That simple gesture was a vindication, especially after being told by some that I had no place in veterans' mental health battles.

IN THE EARLY days of OSISS's formation the Canadian Forces surgeon general was Lise Mathieu.* We spoke several times at NDHQ, and she was very supportive of my work. On one occasion, she informed me that certain people in the chain of command were obsessed with discovering who was faking PTSD. Something she said at the time really stuck with me, and I would repeat it over the years. She said that it

---

* Among other things, the surgeon general is the head of health matters for the Canadian Armed Forces, as well as an advisor to the minister of national defence and the chief of the defence staff.

was surprising that statistics showed somewhere around 3 per cent of people diagnosed with PTSD were faking the condition, yet people were focused on *that* group, while the other 97 per cent genuinely needed help. She believed that it was important to focus on this overwhelming majority. It was empowering to hear that kind of statement from the head of medical services for the Canadian Forces, a sign that things were slowly changing for the better.

During another conversation, in the fall of 2001, General Mathieu suggested that I meet with the psychiatrist I'd had appointments with a few years earlier; she thought it would be a good idea to get his advice about mental health matters. She was unaware that I'd already met with him and felt he was uncooperative, so I politely played along out of appreciation for her support. When our chat ended, I tried to look him up in the DND network, but oddly I was unable to find him, even after trying numerous spellings of his name. Frustrated, I called General Mathieu's office hoping someone there might be able to help. A young officer on the other end of the phone did his best to maintain a serious and professional tone as he informed me that I wouldn't find the doctor under his own name because he used the alias "Jean-Luc Picard." After asking around, I learned that Jean-Luc Picard was the captain of the Starship Enterprise from *Star Trek*. In an attempt to stop people from contacting him—a rather odd thing for a psychiatrist to do—he used a code name to ensure only a select few knew his email.

After hanging up the phone I pondered the bizarre nature of what I'd just learned before sending "Jean-Luc Picard" an email. A week later I drove up to CFB Borden, about an hour north of Toronto, and listened for two hours as Dr. Picard pontificated about what he felt were significant facts. The first half of his monologue focused on his belief that PTSD was exaggerated in many cases, while the second had him trying to wow me with his understanding of the complexities of the brain. It was clear to me that he didn't understand a single thing about what I was trying to do. He wished me luck nonetheless, and I left his office with nothing tangible except a book he lent me on the creation of Alcoholics Anonymous.

A few years later, in 2004, when the OSISS program was up and running, Jim Jamieson and I organized a meeting with Dr. Picard. Its purpose was to try to make amends, build bridges, and foster greater co-operation between clinical and non-clinical mental health workers. Some military physicians still felt uneasy about formally referring their patients to OSISS, largely because they were looking at things through a medical prism and didn't see what we were doing as "evidence-based medicine," despite the fact that I made it clear we provided a *non-clinical* form of support. Jim and I wanted Dr. Picard's help to remedy this situation.

As per usual things went nowhere fast. Dr. Picard was extremely resistant to the idea of even *potentially* referring patients to OSISS. He kept referring to "criteria" and citing doctor-patient confidentiality, even though we never even suggested that peer supporters be given the names of psychiatrists' patients. At the end of the meeting I proposed that perhaps clinicians could just keep OSISS business cards in their desks and, if things went well during a therapy session, casually hand one to their patient so as to make them aware of the program; that way, patients could make up their own mind about whether they'd like to avail themselves of peer support. But even a soft referral was too much for Dr. Picard, and in the end he seemed to view our request as an encroachment on physicians' territory. I learned down the road from a psychiatrist friend, Dr. Don Richardson, who at that time worked as a consultant for Veterans Affairs, that many clinicians initially felt that peer support coordinators were too ill to help others. The general consensus was that they would either be hurting themselves or making things worse for their peers. I could understand their reluctance, but in some cases this went beyond just concern for patients. And as it turned out, peer support worked.

Later in 2004, General Couture was summoned to Parliament Hill to discuss PTSD with a parliamentary standing committee on national defence. He invited General Lise Mathieu, Dr. Picard, and myself to the meeting as well. We were told to arrive at his office an hour before the proceedings, then head across Wellington Street to Parliament, where we would be screened by security. As a major with only a high school diploma, I felt rather intimidated knowing that I'd be in the presence of a psychiatrist, a two-star general, and the military's surgeon general.

When I arrived, Dr. Picard was already sitting, speaking with General Mathieu. I nodded to them both as they stood up to greet me, and then we all sat and stared at the floor in silence. Dr. Picard had always used his concern for patients and the "lack of evidence" about peer support's effectiveness as a way to passive-aggressively denigrate the OSISS program. Now, a few years into OSISS's existence, when it was clear that the program worked, I took the opportunity to chide him in front of the surgeon general. I broke the silence in the room by leaning towards him and inquiring in a lofty tone whether he wanted to ask me how my peer supporters—many of whom were also patients of his—were doing. Playing along, he asked me to tell him. I replied pointedly, "They're doing just fine, doctor, they're doing just fine." Tension pervaded the room for the next few minutes, and it was only broken by the happy-go-lucky General Couture emerging from his office and rallying us for our trip to Parliament Hill.

IN THE SUMMER of 2002 I was still working under David Wrather, managing the OSISS program, when I was posted back to Ottawa. A lot had happened over the past few years—personally, professionally, and in a more general sense, geopolitically. Less than a year had passed since the September 11 terrorist attacks; the war in Afghanistan was heating up, and members of the Third Battalion of the Princess Patricia's Canadian Light Infantry were about to return home after sustaining four dead and eight wounded in the infamous Tarnak Farm incident of April 17, 2002. On that day a U.S. fighter pilot accidentally dropped a 500-pound bomb on his Canadian allies. The four soldiers killed were the first Canadian battlefield deaths since the war began, and the first during a war since Canadians fought in Korea in the early 1950s. Afghanistan was a tough environment, even at the best of times, but since our country hadn't seen war casualties for decades, I sensed that they would hit our troops hard.

By this point OSISS was gathering steam, and I was personally supporting a number of affected soldiers. Hearing various stories and thinking about my own experience in 1995, when I collapsed at my front door upon returning from Rwanda, I started to ponder how we might best help our troops to reintegrate once they returned from Afghanistan. In the 1990s, we often scattered soldiers to the winds right after they returned (especially the reservists). This was a recipe for disaster since it gave soldiers no time to decompress, to mull over experiences with comrades, or have their mental fitness properly assessed by professionals.

I was also influenced by an article by a British surgeon who served during the 1982 Falklands War. The author observed fewer cases of PTSD among the marines, who slowly sailed back to Britain, compared to the airborne troops, who were flown directly home. He theorized that the slow return, which gave soldiers time to unwind and seek solace from comrades, served as a protective factor against future psychological casualties. Combined with my own experiences, and the stories I'd heard from OSISS clients, the article was enough to convince me of the need for change. I emailed a short proposal to General Couture stating my belief in the need to slow down the repatriation and reintegration of Canadian troops.

Unbeknownst to me, Colonel Pat Stogran, the commander of the Princess Patricia's Third Battalion, had made the same request to the deputy chief of the defence staff through his own chain of command. I'd never met Stogran, but his simultaneous request meant that the idea for an alternative way to bring troops home had occurred to us both. General Couture sent my note to the surgeon general at the same time that he received Stogran's idea from the deputy chief. That was enough to convince him of the need for what would later become known as "third location decompression" (TLD). A task force was soon appointed, which met on a regular basis to put together a coherent TLD program for Canada's Afghanistan mission. The TLD program involved sending returning troops on a short (usually three-day) trip to the balmy island of Cyprus, where they were given time to relax, unwind with comrades, and attend both mandatory and elective briefings on health and reintegration. Although some troops used the time to simply get intoxicated after a long and stressful tour, and there were occasional disciplinary problems, overall the TLD program was very well received since it accomplished what it set out to do.

During the program's planning stages, around May 2002, I was invited to a meeting headed by a representative of the deputy chief of the defence staff. The meeting was attended by Dr. Picard, Henry Matheson, the Canadian Force's head of social work, and Dr. Mark Zamorski, an epidemiologist. We discussed the TLD concept for a few hours, and when the floor was opened up attendees began voicing their opinions. Although I was at the table, it was clear that my opinion wouldn't carry the same weight as the other participants' because I wasn't a doctor. Throughout the discussion I kept hearing words to the effect that there was no evidence that TLD would make any difference for returning troops. When it was my turn, I therefore decided to flip the argument on its head. Addressing my comments mainly to Drs. Picard and Zamorski, I pleaded: show me the evidence from the medical literature that says it *won't* work; if there is none, while I appreciate that you don't want to use our soldiers as guinea pigs, we need to innovate here. I then reiterated that it was very unhealthy for a soldier to be in a war zone one minute, and then bouncing a baby on his knee the next.

Evidence is certainly important, and if there was evidence to show that TLD was harmful I would've been the first person to stand against it. But a lack of evidence proving something works doesn't mean that it shouldn't be attempted, especially when the current system has been proven to be broken or ineffective. I spent the next few minutes telling part of the story of my return from Rwanda, mainly to bring some emotion into what was otherwise a very mundane and sterile meeting. I believe that in their rush to worship at the temple of evidence-based medicine, policy-makers and physicians sometimes forget that if we never tried anything new we would have far fewer innovations. Somewhere, sometime, someone has to be the first to try something, even if there aren't any preceding studies to draw from.

As usual, Dr. Picard looked at me with a mixture of apathy and condescension for my having dared to suggest something without a medical degree attached to my name. Dr. Zamorski, for his part, was not against the idea per se, but because he was somewhat stuck in the statistical-analysis box he couldn't fathom the idea working without a pile of studies stating so. But much to Picard's chagrin, the TLD program went forward anyway. Retrospectively, I get the impression that General Couture was moving forward with TLD regardless; the meeting was probably intended as a debate to make sure the program was effectively implemented. But either way, TLD proved to be a success. Soldiers returning from a tough Afghanistan tour were given time to shed their combat boots in favour of flip-flops, and they were allowed the time to let their minds readjust to life outside of a war zone.

A decade later, in 2012, Dr. Zamorski published a paper with Dr. Bryan Garber in *Military Medicine* that evaluated how soldiers returning from Afghanistan felt about TLD. Unsurprisingly (to me at least), not only did 95 per cent of the study's respondents agree that "some form of TLD is a good idea," the paper also concluded that "Canadian Forces members saw value in the TLD program" and "believed that the program had its intended effect of making the reintegration process easier for them."* Eventually, I was also able to convince the powers that be to include OSISS peer supporters in the TLD program. Their inclusion meant that soldiers could opt to participate in an informal session with veterans to discuss the trials and tribulations of reintegration and to learn about what OSISS had to offer should they ever require help in the future.

On a personal level, I heard from a plethora of soldiers over the ensuing years that receiving mental health briefings and speaking with OSISS peer supporters convinced them to seek medical help a lot earlier than they would have, had the TLD program not existed. For me, these stories were another reminder that if we never try anything new we will forever spin our wheels while fresh ideas pass right in front of us.

---

* Those interested in knowing more about TLDs can consult Garber and Zamorski's paper, which is listed in the bibliographical note at the back of this book.

IN THE FALL of 2002, when OSISS had been officially operating for about six months, my peer supporters and I encountered numerous unforeseen challenges as we ironed out the kinks. My first four peer supporters were already meeting with veterans and providing them with much-needed help, but I learned early on that, unlike clinical meetings, which take place in offices and hospitals, peer support meetings happen in various settings. The preferred way my supporters organized chats was the same method used by Canadians for decades: "Let's go for coffee." Unfortunately, they were using personal funds, and although one coffee wasn't going to break the bank, when they met with three or more people per week the costs quickly added up. No one complained, but when I saw a pattern developing I realized that something needed to be done to ensure all those coffees and sandwiches weren't being paid for out of the supporters' pockets.

The DND had a hospitality form that had to be filled out whenever money was being spent on, well, hospitality. Its main purpose was to ensure that public servants weren't spending taxpayers' money on wining and dining friends or family. Usually one filled out hospitality forms when entertaining dignitaries, but in my case, they were to ensure that peer supporters had an informal place to meet their "clients." So I filled out the forms and sent them off, and a few weeks later David Wrather gave me the bad news—they had been denied. This was surprising: I felt this was a justified use of money, and Dave had been very supportive of my endeavours, but ultimately he didn't have the final say. I even reapplied with different wording, but was denied again.

Frustrated, I eventually decided to try another route. I sat down at my desk and drafted a letter to the president of Tim Hortons outlining OSISS's mandate and what my peer supporters did to help injured soldiers. I asked if he could provide gift cards or some other way for my employees to avoid paying out of pocket for their work. Serendipitously, Dave came by my desk that day to ask how things were going. When I mentioned my latest strategy he said it was a good idea, but asked me to let him run it by the people who approved hospitality funding before I sent off my request; he wanted to make the case that it would be highly embarrassing for the DND if Tim Hortons had to sponsor those helping injured veterans. Within a week, the bureaucrats, now worried about potential embarrassment, approved my request. I allowed my peer supporters a very reasonable amount of funding per month, and to the best of my knowledge it was never abused.

My right-hand man at OSISS was Jim Woodley, a former chief warrant officer with the Princess Patricia's. As an ex-CWO and career manager, he knew the system inside and out, and was adroit at understanding how to handle military and government bureaucracies. One week in the late fall of 2003, Jim went to Halifax to liaise with OSISS support staff in Nova Scotia. While there he learned from our peer supporter on the ground about a soldier under care for an operational stress injury who'd skipped town, leaving his wife, a stay-at-home mom of several kids, with no money. It was the end of November, and with the furnace in her house lacking oil and the heat turned off, the situation was going from bad to worse. Ultimately, the case ended up being a perfect example of the corollary benefits of having a peer support program. After all, it wasn't the doctor's job to find the missing patient. Indeed, he wasn't really a "missing" person at all: he'd simply taken off.

Jim was scheduled to fly home, but we knew he couldn't leave things as they were. He had the corporate credit card with him, and we had a contingency fund at the Casualty Support office to bail out people in dire straits; but the paperwork and approval usually took a day or two, and the man who oversaw this process was in meetings all day. I asked Jim if he had room on his personal credit card to pay for the furnace oil; I would ensure that he was paid back from either the contingency fund or my own personal bank account. Jim went ahead and paid, but unsurprisingly the finance people at Casualty Support gave me a hard time, saying we needed to follow the proper rules in such situations. This pushback was another reminder of how some in the DND were so obsessed with following procedures to the letter that they forgot why those procedures existed in the first place. Protocols and procedures became, for many, an end in and of themselves, rather than means for helping *human beings*. A family needed heat in their home and it couldn't wait—plain and simple.

Later that fall, I received a phone call from the mother of a young reservist who lived on Montreal's South Shore. She was beside herself, yelling into the phone that her son was in the backyard tying a rope to a tree and preparing to hang himself. I knew there was no time to lose. I told her to let him know that I wanted to speak with him. She relayed my message, but to no avail. After a few minutes of trying to calm her down I worried that her son was going to complete the act while we were on the phone, so I told her sternly, "Go outside and tell him the colonel wants to speak with him—now!" She obliged and went to deliver my message. My demonstration of authority seemed to snap him out of it, and he finally came to the phone. I told him to stop what he was doing, explained that there were other options, and gave him the number of our peer support coordinator in Montreal, who later got him the help he needed. His mother was understandably shaken up that day, but happy that her son had received help. Later, after I called to ensure the situation was sorted, I took a deep breath and leaned back in my desk chair, wondering how the situation would've turned out if I had said any number of other things.

Less than an hour after the call, a padre (Canadian Forces chaplain) who'd overheard part of my conversation from his adjacent cubicle came over to speak with me. He sat down and said in a gentle and calm way, as padres do, that I was engaged in very difficult work, and that he was worried about the impact on my own health. I chuckled and told him that I had no problem dealing with a mother whose son was about to kill himself—what I found most difficult and stressful was the fucking bureaucracy I was forced to work within. He looked at me for a moment, and then we both started laughing.

By early 2003 OSISS had expanded to about ten peer supporters. Then, as now, peer supporters often encountered soldiers in the midst of being discharged from the Canadian Forces or lost in a bureaucratic labyrinth while trying to obtain help. In those situations we always did our best to help them sort things out and, if they were being released, prepare them for life as a civilian. The process could be quite frustrating, particularly since at times it seemed like government bureaucrats handled files as if the information contained within didn't reflect actual human beings. In the military especially, which is obsessed with soldiers' ability to deploy at a moment's notice, this produced a mentality that if someone wasn't doing well they weren't worth the paper their file was printed on. One example of this attitude was the sending of intent-to-release forms (essentially military pink slips) to soldiers in December, right before Christmas. David Wrather and I eventually convinced the Military Careers Administration to send them no later than November. Apparently, it hadn't occurred to anyone that sending these forms right before Christmas was a sure-fire way to ruin a family's holidays and make a bad situation worse.

On one occasion I discovered that a soldier we were supporting was suicidal and undergoing very intense psychotherapy. One of my peer supporters also got wind that the directorate was planning to send the man a pink slip. We knew it wouldn't be long before the letter was reviewed by the director, signed, and sent, so we arranged an emergency meeting with him to discuss things. Our intent was not to convince him not to sign the letter, but simply to ask him to hold off for a little while until we could ensure the man's mental state was less fragile.

David Wrather and I arrived at NDHQ at about 3:00 p.m. We located the director's office, but he was nowhere to be found, so we waited. He showed up about forty-five minutes later, and after some brief pleasantries we stated our case. He quickly made it clear that he wasn't budging, and that he was worried that if he started making exceptions the release process would be held up. We pressed our case for several minutes, but it was obvious we weren't making any headway: the director kept looking at his watch, the universal sign for "I'm done with this conversation." Then something stunning occurred. While Dave was in the midst of speaking the director got up, walked around to the front of his desk, grabbed his coat from the coat rack, and began to walk out the door. Somewhat shocked, Dave asked where he was going, to which he received the matter-of-fact reply, "I've got a bus to catch." Then he just left.

Dave and I looked at each other in disbelief, shocked by the insensitivity and rudeness we'd just witnessed. He could have told us that he was taking his wife out for dinner, or simply that he would think about it and get back to us. Instead, he blatantly lied. That was just one example of the kind of obstruction and indifference mental health advocates encountered when trying to modify how the military treated injured soldiers.

Co-morbidity—the fancy medical term for multiple conditions presenting in a patient at the same time—is common among soldiers with mental injuries. It isn't hard to find a soldier diagnosed with PTSD who also has, say, depression or a substance abuse problem. When someone is unaware that they have a mental health problem it's easy for the troubles to keep piling on. I can recall several occasions when a soldier with PTSD who'd also developed an alcohol problem was caught driving under the influence. While this type of infraction is already serious in a civilian context, it carries even graver consequences for a soldier: those *medically* released from the military are entitled to an indexed pension and benefits (assuming they've been in the military long enough, of course). Those released for disciplinary reasons, on the other hand, are not.

The medical release process often took up to a year, and in that time a lot could happen. As soldiers mentally adjusted to the idea of life outside the military, for some the only career and world they'd ever known, they often felt overwhelmed. Just like in the civilian realm, people cope with illness and change in different ways, and some soldiers decided that the best coping mechanism was alcohol. When a soldier abusing alcohol was caught doing illegal activities, like driving drunk, the career directorate was informed. Very quickly afterward the reason for release would often change from medical reasons to "conduct unbecoming," or some other kind of dishonourable discharge. We certainly weren't advocating for lighter penalties for drunk drivers: I, along with everyone else at OSISS, felt offending soldiers should be charged and given the same penalties as everyone else. What we *were* asking for was that the military not strip them of release benefits. My argument was this: if we were releasing someone anyway, we shouldn't take away their benefits at the last minute because of a charge during the last year of their career. Otherwise, we should review *all* the files and treat those who misbehaved early in their careers the same way.

The fact is that a lot of soldiers with substance abuse issues are coping with multiple problems, including mental ones. And yet, as far as I'm concerned, the manner in which a lot of these soldiers were being released was deliberately punitive. Most of them were either too angry or too sick to advocate for themselves, so Dave or I, or OSISS peer supporters, sometimes advocated on their behalf. I tried to avoid such activities because I knew that, strictly speaking, they weren't part of OSISS's role, but when dealing with human beings who were being treated so unfairly it was difficult at times to remain entirely objective.

IN THE WAKE of the 2002 friendly fire incident in Afghanistan, it became obvious that we were involved in a mission that would have a significant impact, not just on Canadian soldiers, but on their families, too. As Canadian participation in the war increased, and especially after plans were made to send more troops during the 2004–05 period, military casualties, both mental and physical, were expected to increase

Considering what was going on overseas, and especially the impact these developments would have on military families, I decided to look into the possibility of launching another component for the OSISS program, one that could help families. Families were sometimes left in the lurch, even when the military claimed to have their back.

In 2004, for example, the Veterans Affairs opened a clinic in Winnipeg. Shortly thereafter I received a call from a soldier's spouse, a woman who'd been heavily impacted by her husband's mental turmoil. She had sought treatment at the Winnipeg clinic but was turned away, despite Veterans Affairs proudly proclaiming on its pamphlets that the clinic served veterans and their families. I made some phone calls to get to the bottom of things, and was told that family members were welcome to attend veterans' therapy sessions, but they weren't able to receive treatment themselves. Enraged, I told a few unlucky bureaucrats that people's health was in the balance and that they should immediately change the wording of their pamphlets. Such shameful situations confirmed that families needed more than what was out there.

After some initial research I spoke with Dave Wrather, who agreed that providing soldiers' families with better support was a good idea. With his blessing I commissioned a study of families of those suffering from PTSD. I wanted to discover what their needs were, and whether they felt they could benefit from a support program.

The post-study report showed a correlation between spouses being exposed to military members' health troubles and negative long-term effects on their own health. It also concluded that family members needed support and treatment if they developed a mental health condition of their own from months or years of dealing with family turmoil. Lastly, it affirmed the need for education about what operational stress injuries are, so that at the very least families could understand what was happening with their loved ones. Ultimately, the report was a way to convince Veterans Affairs and the DND to invest more money in OSISS and extend peer support services to family members. To both departments' credit, and with some degree of surprise on my part, the program was given the green light in a few months' time, probably because they knew the fallout from Afghanistan would only grow with time.

Though I knew that soldiers' deaths in Afghanistan would hit families hard, I also knew that the numbers wouldn't be big enough to warrant employing full-time bereavement supporters. I decided that the best way forward was to leverage volunteers—those who'd been through bereavement themselves and could help others face such a difficult time. Since that type of approach didn't require OSISS budget increases and approvals, I took it upon myself to make it happen. Things progressed well, but as is common in big organizations, some members felt that their territory was being encroached upon.

One day in early 2005, a padre who worked at the Casualty Support Administration got wind that I was adding a bereavement component to the OSISS program, and he asked to speak with me in his office. When we sat down he went on at length about the complexity of bereavement, and he said that I should be very careful, since bereaved widows and widowers are very fragile. Judging by his tone, and the way he kept referring to the traditional role of padres, he seemed to be implying that I was in over my head. Although he was a very nice man who felt he was doing the right thing, he was essentially telling me, albeit subtly, to back off, that I'd stepped on his toes. I understood his point of view, but I also felt like traditional approaches had in many ways failed to adapt to the changing nature of military operations and new understandings of mental health. No one owns bereavement, and I was a bit frustrated that he seemed to see the program as competition, rather than as a helpful adjunct to the important work padres do. At any rate, the whole conversation felt a bit condescending. I thanked him for his advice but went ahead regardless.

While the program was shaping up I decided to look at the most recent casualties list and find the families that had lost a loved one. My goal was to gather the names of about a dozen families whom I could consult; I wanted to know if peer support had any relevance for people in their situation. I also felt that this was the best way to canvass for volunteers who could help shape the program and support those in need. Finding these families was a difficult task, though, since once a soldier dies their contact information is tightly controlled by the DND—not just anyone can call a widow or bereaved parents out of the blue. My search therefore involved a lot of emails, phone calls, and networking across various chains of command in all three branches of the military. In the end this took several months.

But finally, the time came in the early spring of 2005 to call the families and see who was willing to speak with me. I was quite nervous. They'd been through a lot, and I didn't know what their feelings were toward the DND and the military, the organizations that ultimately led to their family member's death. But I did know that their input would be crucial, so I took a deep breath, began at the top of the list, and started dialing. Each time someone answered I introduced myself, thanked them for speaking with me, and explained what my goal was. I also invited them to meet with me in person, if they were willing. To my surprise, everyone unreservedly said yes. I'd been told by the aforementioned padre that they might hang up, break down, or be hostile, but instead they were eager to help. The people I spoke with took the project on as their cause, their way to ensure that others in a similar situation would have the support they didn't.

Once I received their agreement, a meeting date was set. Our gathering took place in Edmonton on May 31, 2005. I had my team with me, including Jim Woodley, my national coordinator, and Sophie Richard, a social worker I hired to manage OSISS's family peer support component. Sophie was my iron fist in a velvet glove, as they say; she had a knack for organization and could firmly but delicately manage disparate groups of people. My idea was to use the meeting to get things rolling before handing the program over to her for further development.

In attendance at the meeting were Marley Leger, Tina Beerenfenger, Belinda Naismith, Deanne Nichols, Brian Isfeld, Jim Davis, Julie Selby, Gwen Saunders, Mellissa Lesquire, Jacinthe Couture, and Heather Dillon. After brief introductions I explained the concept of peer support, and I asked if they felt it would be of use to grieving families. Without hesitation they all said yes. When push came to shove, they explained, it wasn't the padre, the assisting officer, or even extended family members that they found most helpful after their loved one's death—it was those who'd been through the same experience. Indeed, they related several stories about serendipitous chats between grieving families, and how those chance encounters allowed them to, for the first time, speak with someone who they felt *truly* understood what they were going through.

I was still concerned, though: since OSISS dealt with mental health, were they comfortable being associated with what was still a taboo subject? I wanted to be sure that they were clear on what OSISS did, and how their association with it might be viewed by friends and colleagues. They all looked rather confused. After a few moments of silence Deanne Nichols politely asked me, "What do you think bereavement is?" Several others then related their battles with depression and anxiety after losing their loved one.

For them, it was self-evident that bereavement and mental health went hand-in-hand; they therefore had absolutely no problem being associated with OSISS. I felt a bit foolish for not knowing what was obvious to everyone else in the room, but this was a reminder that even after several years of working with OSISS I still had a lot to learn about mental health. Others in attendance related how military family resource centres did an important job, but that their services were more on the "soft" side—things like barbecues and daycare. Facing bereavement required an additional type of support. By the end of our day-long meeting, it was unanimous: everyone was on board to be the new program's first volunteers.

When my team returned to Ottawa, Sophie began looking for an organization that could complement basic peer support training, someone to help volunteers further understand the bereavement process and what complications might arise as a result. Each person handles grief differently, after all. Some feel the constant need to talk about their loss; others simply withdraw from social situations altogether. We felt it was important that peer supporters understood the varying paths people take on their journey to recovery. We pieced together a training program with a strong bereavement training component, and within a few months our first volunteer cohort was trained and ready to help. The HOPE (Helping Our Peer by Providing Empathy) program was born. It continues to this day under Sophie's excellent guidance.

ALTHOUGH I WAS successful from 2001 to 2005 in helping to implement new programs for mentally injured veterans and their families, my job as OSISS manager was increasingly at risk as I challenged the DND bureaucracy, and from about 2003 onwards my star slowly began to fall. In 2004 a new minister of national defence, Bill Graham, took over. I was given the task of writing an extensive briefing note for him on the state of affairs for soldiers with PTSD and how the military managed mental health issues. The process of preparing and editing that note was, quite frankly, ridiculous. I was the lead author, but not the only one, and I had no idea that I was going to be up against a spin-doctoring exercise by the surgeon general's office.

I wrote the first version and showed it to the DND stakeholders, and then the editing process began. From the moment the first draft left my hands a conscious, calculated sanitization effort was undertaken, largely to excise any negative assessments. Very quickly I felt like the document had taken on a life of its own and was no longer mine. By the eighth or ninth version, about three weeks into the process, I told my boss, Lieutenant-Colonel Gerry Blais, that the edited note was inaccurate and untruthful. I asked for my name to be removed: I wanted no part of it. That move was politically incorrect, and it turned out to be one of the factors that led to my demise as OSISS manager.

The other factor that made me unpopular was my decision, in 2005, to send a very frank email to then senator Roméo Dallaire about the New Veterans Charter, which was being discussed in Parliament that year. In my message I implored Dallaire not to vote for the new charter. Devised by Prime Minister Paul Martin and his Liberal Party in 2005, the charter certainly did a lot of good, especially by updating legislation about veterans' benefits, programs, and pensions enacted back in 1919, just after the end of the First World War. But it also had a few major flaws.

For example, one of the issues OSISS and I felt strongest about was the new lump-sum payment for ill or injured vets, which did away with the previous lifelong payment scheme. Our issue was simple: how could we in our right minds give $150,000 or more to a soldier with PTSD, depression, and a substance abuse problem? In our materialistic culture that kind of money could be spent in a matter of days by someone looking for a short-term fix to a long-term problem. And it often was. Once the money was gone you still had an injured vet with no more money coming in to help them get on their feet again. The lump-sum payment struck me as an obvious, and cynical, attempt at offloading long-term financial responsibility for injured veterans, and I couldn't abide by it.

Veterans Affairs countered that providing money on a monthly basis was paternalistic, that it amounted to managing veterans' finances for them. But in my mind the evils of the lump-sum payment far outweighed any downsides of a payment in perpetuity. What was worse, I wondered: appearing paternalistic and having a veteran taken care of financially for life? or *appearing* magnanimous and having an injured veteran penniless after less than a year?

OSISS and other veterans' advocates rightly predicted that the lump-sum payment would be one of the new charter's biggest shortfalls, as various newspaper articles and academic studies went on to show. And so I made the decision to email Senator Dallaire. Instead of reading my email and taking it under advisement, however, he made the unintentional mistake of forwarding it to Veterans Affairs, to confirm if what I said was true. He certainly didn't intend to get me in trouble, as I found out during a later discussion, but in the end that email cost me my job. Infuriated by my message to Dallaire, the powers that be at Veterans Affairs called the DND, and the next thing I knew I was posted out—essentially fired—from my job. My email was an embarrassment to my boss, a vice admiral, and when powerful people get embarrassed someone gets the axe. I had refused to toe the party line on several occasions throughout my career, and it finally cost me.

As a sad addendum to that chapter of my life, General Couture, by then recently retired, was killed in a snowmobiling accident in January 2006. He was just fifty-six; as they say, only the good die young. Shortly after his death, I went with two peer supporters to visit his widow, Jacinthe, at their home in Lac Saint-Jean. Before we left she insisted that I see the general's den in the basement. Unsurprisingly, the entire basement was filled with the various plaques and awards the general had received over his many years of service. Jacinthe told us that her husband cherished all of them, but he was particularly fond of a painting of an injured soldier on weathered wood that I'd given him in thanks for his support in OSISS's creation. Instead of placing it with the other awards and recognitions, he'd put it on the stairwell leading down to his den so that he could see it every time he walked up and down the stairs.

I still get choked up when I think about that. Several years later Tom Martineau, an OSISS regional coordinator, said it best when he told me that General Couture had provided me with the soil in which to sow the seeds of OSISS.

Chapter 7

AFGHANISTAN AND BEYOND

By late August 2006 I had been removed from OSISS over my outspokenness about the New Veterans Charter's shortcomings. I was working a boring desk job at NDHQ helping to determine if Canada could play a more prominent training role in NATO, when it came to my attention that NATO wanted a Canadian lieutenant-colonel to work at its Regional Command South headquarters in Afghanistan. My son David was heading off to university the following summer, and I didn't want to leave Julie and Veronique to deal with the harsh Cantley winter, so I figured it would be beneficial for everyone if I could get my tour over with by summer 2007. So I immediately went to my boss, Chris Henderson, and said, "I'm your man for the job." He agreed, and by November I started pre-deployment training, which involved, among other things, weapons training, mine and explosive ordnance awareness, and cultural sensitivity training. A few months later I was ready to go.

On a cold and snowy day in January 2007 I hugged David and Veronique, who were now old enough to understand the war in Afghanistan. They looked a little like deer in the headlights as we said goodbye. Even though I would not be in a combat role, they were still worried. After saying an emotional goodbye to the kids, Julie took me to the train station in Ottawa, and we prepared to part ways, as we'd done several times before. On the platform I picked up my bags, quickly kissed her goodbye, and walked away without looking back; it was always easiest that way. I boarded the train and watched the snow falling outside as I made my way toward Belleville, the next stop before my arrival at CFB Trenton.

A long time had passed since I was on an overseas operation, so I was slightly apprehensive. I also knew that the war in Afghanistan was a brutal struggle with no clear-cut way to measure if the good guys were winning. Indeed, in some instances you couldn't even tell who the good guys were. I also had a feeling of guilt in the pit of my stomach as I thought about yet again leaving Julie and the kids while I went on another military operation. But as the train picked up speed I tried to put those thoughts out of my head for the moment. Sleep is a precious commodity during any tour, and I knew I should stock up while I could.

When I got to Trenton three hours later I checked my luggage and boarded a flight bound for Germany. There wasn't a single empty seat on the plane as we waited on the tarmac, but Old Man Winter had decided it wasn't our day to leave. After close to an hour of waiting it became clear that the amount of snow on the ground and in the air had made it impossible to leave. I heard lots of muffled grumbling as the plane was unloaded, bags were returned to their owners, and we were issued sleeping quarters for the night. Disappointed but tired and ready for sleep, I went to my room and crashed for the night.

In the morning there were more delays. The plane didn't get off the ground until close to lunchtime, and by the time we arrived in Germany it was the middle of the night. Departing once again from Germany, the plane stopped at some obscure place (I can't recall the name) to refuel before another long flight to Dubai. Once there, we took a bus to a military base for another overnight stay before our flight to Afghanistan the next morning. I was jet-lagged but slept like a baby after so many uncomfortable hours on the plane—and this despite my knowledge that the next flight was taking me to one of the most dangerous places on earth.

Early the next morning we were issued our rifle and gear ("bombed up," in military lingo) before waiting yet again for our flight to Afghanistan, which didn't leave until that night. Most of the soldiers passed the hours by checking their equipment, looking for familiar faces, and shooting the breeze with those who'd previously been deployed to Afghanistan. By that point, instead of being scared, I was more curious about how this tour would compare with the others I'd done. Thinking about past experiences made the time go quickly, and before I knew it I was on yet another Hercules transport bound for Kandahar.

Once the plane was up in the air I looked around at all the faces: it was immediately obvious who'd done multiple tours. One young corporal across from me was armed to the teeth, and his combat clothing was almost entirely faded from the sun. He looked vacant and weary, in the way that hardened soldiers often do. I could tell that this wasn't his first time at the rodeo. I hadn't deployed in a long time, but because of my own experience with an OSI, and my time working with so many injured soldiers in the OSISS program, I could spot with some degree of accuracy who was struggling. You didn't have to be concerned about the soldiers who looked anxious; it was the ones whose faces looked flat and lifeless that were usually at risk of developing a mental health issue. Whenever I glanced up from my Sudoku puzzles and scanned the plane, my eyes always settled on that young corporal, with his archetypal thousand-yard stare and faded camouflage. His image is seared in my mind, and I've always wondered what happened to him in the subsequent months and years.

When we landed at Kandahar Airfield the first hangar I saw was riddled with bullet holes. It had been the site of a December 2001 battle between U.S. Marines and Taliban forces, and no one had bothered to fix the damage. We were marshalled for a welcome briefing, which included such warnings as "no sex on the base," and "no drinking on the base," etc. That pep talk was a bit awkward and embarrassing for a group of adults, some of whom had thirty years' experience in the military. We were essentially being spoken to like teenagers. All I could think was, "the army never changes."

Over the course of that day we were given more briefings and training before we were brought to our temporary quarters after midnight. It had rained heavily that day, and because the ground was packed so tightly, like cement, water didn't drain very well. When a group of us got to our quarters I watched with anger as our gear was carelessly thrown off a large truck into puddles of water. It wasn't even my first full day in Afghanistan and already my gear was wet and muddy. I picked up my bags and walked into the sleeping quarters only to discover that I was to sleep at the top of a bunk bed; the bottom bunk had been given to a private. It's not that I was too good to sleep in the same room as a subordinate, but I was upset because such logistical laziness created an awkward situation: non-commissioned members sometimes feel constrained and nervous around officers. I went to sleep frustrated at what I'd seen thus far, but I tried my best to maintain my composure for the days ahead.

My first full day was taken up with more lectures and briefings. Thankfully, on one of our breaks, a captain who was going to be working for me, André Salloum, came and introduced himself. André was a kind and likeable fellow who knew how intimidating it was to arrive in Kandahar alone, instead of with a unit. He brought me to my office, introduced me to the staff, and helped me get acclimatized to my new surroundings. After listening to condescending briefings, André's kindness was a welcome respite, and he was a great help to me as I tried to find a groove during my first week in theatre.

I was in charge of a small staff and a few Afghan translators. Our job was to oversee communications with the local and international media—a safe job but still a stressful one thanks to the Internet and the twenty-four-seven news cycle. I was replacing a British major who seemed like a decent enough guy, but who had an ego bigger than the largest truck on the base. From day one he didn't like me, partially, it seemed, because I outranked him, and partially because he had that "what do these Canadian colonials know?" kind of attitude often (still) prevalent in British officer circles.

AS I WALKED into the office about two weeks into my tour André told me not to go anywhere because the Canadians were about to kill someone. I was perplexed by his statement, so I asked for clarification. He explained: a Canadian Light Armoured Vehicle, or LAV as we call them, had broken down on its way back to base. The procedure under these circumstances was for the soldiers to get out, set up a barrier around the LAV—by this point a sitting duck—and wait for a recovery vehicle to tow it out. In the meantime, civilian traffic still went on as usual, but it was necessary for the soldiers guarding the LAV to order vehicles to stop or slow down on approach, to ensure that the driver wasn't a suicide bomber. Unfortunately, due to language differences, cultural misunderstandings, and the universal tendency of some people to panic in stressful situations, civilian drivers would occasionally either fail to stop, or deliberately try to break through the barrier. This is exactly what had occurred. With the accompanying troops now spooked, the stage was set for disaster.

About fifteen minutes later, just as André predicted, we heard over the radio that the Canadians had opened fire. The car's occupants were dead, or, in contemporary military parlance, there'd been "collateral damage." Once again I began to see how a soldier's moral compass can be knocked off balance by the situations encountered in war. I knew that the soldiers who fired on that vehicle—whose occupants turned out not to be carrying any explosives—would always carry the guilt of killing other human beings, even if it was done to protect their fellow soldiers from potential harm. For the rest of their lives, even during times of tranquility, their minds would occasionally be brought back to that brief moment when they had to make that terrible choice to pull the trigger, not knowing whether they were firing on a suicide bomber or an innocent farmer. For some Canadian soldiers, that was daily life in Afghanistan.

During the first few days in theatre new arrivals had to accomplish several tasks, things like zeroing their weapon (aligning the sights) on a firing range, getting paperwork in order, and going to see a travel specialist to book future leaves. Together these tasks were called the "in routine." As part of my in routine I had to sit with a young administration clerk and complete my paperwork. She was a corporal who looked to be in her mid-twenties, and was very smartly dressed. I could tell by her demeanour that she was intelligent and dedicated to her job. We had a good chat as she helped me with ticking boxes and all the other administrative minutiae that goes with being a soldier in the twenty-first century.

About three months later I was getting lunch in the cafeteria when I ran into her again. At first she seemed a bit intimidated because of my rank, but within a few minutes things were comfortable. Almost instantly, however, I could see something about her demeanour was different than when we'd met at the beginning of my tour. When I asked her if anything was wrong she explained that she was anxious: the next day she was going to be part of a convoy heading outside the base. Her primary duties were administrative, and although everyone in the military is expected to be ready to fight if need be, people get acclimatized to their specific job; it sets their expectations for the kind of danger they'll encounter during their daily routine. Her job usually entailed sitting behind a computer and doing paperwork, so going outside the base, where enemy attacks were common, wasn't exactly a welcome task.

We tend to think that infantry troops are the only ones at risk of developing an osi, largely because an entire deployment can sometimes consist of being exposed to danger. But in a way, that exposure can be a protective barrier, too, since it sets their expectations and, to a certain degree, acclimatizes them to risk. Anyone who's seen a gentle-looking, non-macho infantry soldier stoically head off to fight Taliban soldiers will know what this kind of attitude looks like. For a corporal working in administration, on the other hand, going on a convoy mission, getting attacked, and having to shoot enemy combatants is far outside their daily reality. When faced with such a situation, the needle of their moral compass flies all over the place. They know they have a job to do, but they are also worried about what they will face and whether they'll be up to the task. Being scared or uncertain while wearing a military uniform is, in and of itself, seen as a transgression of proper conduct, so some soldiers use up a lot of their courage just trying to appear nonchalant when facing danger or difficult moral decisions.

I never judged someone for developing an OSI, no matter what their background or job, but seeing that clerk so visibly anxious and affected by what the future might hold made me realize that the military needed to cast off the belief that only those who killed Taliban or saw their buddy die were "entitled" to develop mental health problems. A military clerk might be more accustomed to, and indeed trained for, dangerous situations than, say, a civilian, but extreme vigilance and the chemical surge of adrenalin that comes with engaging the enemy aren't part of their routine. On occasion I questioned whether it was in anyone's best interest to have clerks and other administrative staff heading out to fight, since their minds weren't as prepared for the events they might face.

I don't know what happened to the female corporal in question, or how she would've handled a distressing situation, but it was obvious that she was affected by the prospect of stepping so far outside of her comfort zone. Had she encountered mental difficulties, many of her comrades would've looked at her and said something like, "You can't have an OSI, you're only a clerk," or "You only left the base a few times—we were outside the wire the entire time." Culturally, military members decide who is allowed to have an OSI and who isn't, and that determination is often based on how many people you've killed or how many bodies you've seen. But stress and trauma come in many forms, and one person's traumatic situation can be, for some individuals, just another day at work. My conversation with that clerk, and numerous other chats I subsequently had with both soldiers and civilians affected by mental health challenges, allowed me to see the subject through a new lens. We all face different degrees of stress and anxiety, but that doesn't mean that certain types are more legitimate than others, or that some peoples' health challenges are more justified than those of their peers.

I HAD BEEN in Afghanistan for several months when Master Corporal Darrell Priede, a military photographer, arrived to take up a post on my Kandahar staff. At the time most of the fighting was happening outside of Kandahar province, the Canadians' area of responsibility. In May 2007, an American battalion was being flown to Helmand province in an attempt to dislodge the Taliban. On the night of the operation, Corporal Priede and his British counterpart, Corporal Mike Gilyeat (who also worked for me), flew with the Americans as they began a massive air assault. Their job was to capture imagery of the assault.

I remember going to the airhead to see the operation get started. What a sight. The entire air fleet of Regional Command South had been commandeered for what was to be a massive assault on Taliban forces, so the whole tarmac was covered with helicopters from different NATO countries. I spoke briefly with the American battalion commander, and I asked why there were lots of vehicles but so few troops, and he casually responded that they were slowly trickling in; they had to get a coffee at the Tim Hortons first. While our chat continued the number of soldiers swelled, and within minutes the entire area was covered with camouflaged troops, all ready to fight and survive for several days in the field. Most of them stayed standing because they knew that if they sat down the amount of gear on their backs meant they would probably need help getting up again. Off to my left I saw a padre leading about a hundred soldiers in prayer. Soon, loud yelling began to pierce through the drone of the helicopters as troops organized and assembled for departure. In a few minutes they began boarding, and soon after the first wave flew away into the night sky. I remained long enough to watch Priede and Gilyeat head off before retiring to my quarters for the night.

An hour later, there was a knock at my door. The personnel staff officer walked in and informed me that there had been casualties. I went to the office around 1:30 a.m., and my jaw dropped when I realized that it was my two guys, Priede and Gilyeat. They had been riding in a Chinook helicopter with five American soldiers when the Taliban scored a lucky hit with a rocket-propelled grenade. The chopper crashed and all seven people were killed. Of course, casualties weren't an uncommon event in Afghanistan, but never in a hundred years did I think that they'd be soldiers who worked for me.

I spent the next hour trying to piece together exactly what had happened, but when I realized that I wouldn't be able to learn anything until the morning, I went for a walk across the sprawling Kandahar Airfield to clear my head. I was very disturbed, and I knew that my entire staff would be, too, when they got the news the next day. Priede's and Gilyeat's deaths caused a series of memories from Rwanda to flood back into my mind, some of which I hadn't thought about since the 1990s. It had been ten years, and I was in Afghanistan under very different circumstances, but all of the same feelings of guilt, anxiety, and loss arose inside of me and caused my mind to start spinning.

There was nothing I could have done to prevent my subordinates' deaths, but my moral compass nonetheless began flying all over the place. All of the could haves, would haves, and should haves in the world can't stop situations like that from getting to you, making you wonder if you are somehow responsible. The only thing I knew for sure was that two families were going to get phone calls that would change the course of their lives forever. Eventually, while walking past the base's various tents and buildings, I lost track of time, and I suddenly smelled the stench of sewage: in my fugue-like state I'd walked to the far end of the base and was now standing in front of the open-air sewage-treatment facilities. I did my best to collect my thoughts on the long walk back to my sleeping quarters.

While I sat in my office the next morning, still stunned by the previous night's events, a member of the forensic investigation team, a military police sergeant-major, came to see me. He introduced himself and told me that his job was to ensure that Corporal Priede's body was speedily and properly repatriated to his loved ones. When he spoke I could tell from his beleaguered tone of voice that he'd been forced to perform this grim task numerous times already. He also added that, thankfully, Priede, Gilyeat, and the others died quickly and probably didn't feel anything. It was a small bit of consolation, but I was gutted nonetheless.

After the shock subsided, my thoughts immediately drifted to Corporal Priede's family in Canada. When I left for Afghanistan the OSISS HOPE program had been in full swing. Once I knew that Corporal Priede's family had received the tragic news I sent a message to the OSISS team to ensure that they didn't forget to offer their services. Sadly, I was now calling upon the very program I'd helped launch to aid a fallen comrade's family.

Years later Corporal Priede's mother Roxanne became a volunteer for the HOPE bereavement program, and in 2012 she attended the Remembrance Day ceremonies in Ottawa as a Silver Cross Mother. I made sure to meet with her and her husband John during one of their visits to Ottawa, to answer any questions they had about Darrell's death and give them my condolences. One small bit of comfort I got from that sad chapter was the knowledge that at least the program I created was helping the Priede family, who in turn were helping others in similar circumstances.

DAYS WERE LONG in Afghanistan. Most of the time I woke up early in the morning, worked until ten or eleven at night, crashed, and woke up to do it all again the following day. When I needed to decompress I lay on my cot, turned on my iPod, and did some Sudoku puzzles until I was tired. While going through that routine I often found my mind drifting off, to thoughts of a more enjoyable home life after Afghanistan. I kept thinking, hoping: "Things are going to be better when I get back."

Deploying to Rwanda in 1994 changed the dynamic of family life in my house. To be sure, the kids grew up to be just fine—they were everything we could've hoped for—but over the years my marriage slowly eroded. Julie and I still loved one another, but we weren't *in love* anymore. Our household ran smoothly enough, but we both spent most of our time alone. As the saying goes, we were strangers under the same roof. I'll never know for certain if my marriage would've eroded regardless of my time in Rwanda, but the difficulties I faced afterward definitely drove a wedge between us, one that we could never dislodge, no matter how hard we tried. By the time I went to Afghanistan, I had a much better understanding of OSIs and how they affected a marriage, but I still hoped that when I returned things could be fixed. I kept having thoughts that maybe Julie and I could garden together when I got home, or go for walks—anything to bring us closer together again.

In the years between Rwanda and Afghanistan, Julie had found a new identity for herself at the high school where she taught. Kids naturally gravitated to her, and they were willing to share what troubled them at home. Over time she became the school's de facto social worker. She was also a dedicated French teacher who spent many evenings marking at the kitchen table, making sure all of her students finished the class in better shape than when they started. Julie gave everything to her students, and her teaching role became a way to carve out an identity that wasn't tied to me or my problems.

At the same time, I constantly kept busy with numerous home projects. We had several acres of land, so I was always cutting the grass, chopping firewood, taking care of the pool, and maintaining our sugar shack. Essentially, Julie and I kept so busy that the fence between us slowly became a wall, and the wall eventually became impenetrable. Still, I hoped after Afghanistan we could meet on neutral grounds and find the happiness that eluded us.

I RETURNED FROM Afghanistan in the summer of 2007. On the plane ride home I felt gloomy but nonetheless eager to start living life again. I'd come to think of my time in Afghanistan as a pause from the troubles back home, and I hoped that when I returned I'd have another chance to fix things with Julie. I knew that I was the one who'd changed, and therefore the one who needed to try and fit in again. The difficulties I'd faced after Rwanda left me feeling like I couldn't live a so-called normal life, one consisting of grocery lists, barbecues, and talking with extended family about gas prices.

But a few months after I returned it hit me like a ton of bricks: I could never get our old family life back. Veronique, all grown up and waiting to hear back from universities, told us that we had her permission to open any letter from the University of Ottawa. One evening when I got home from work I checked the mail and saw a letter for her. I opened it and, unsurprisingly, it was a letter of acceptance to the university's Telfer School of Business. It felt like a jug of cold water had been thrown in my face. For a few minutes I just stood in the kitchen holding the letter, frozen. The first question that eventually popped into my head was, "Now what?" David was already gone, and Veronique was also about to embark on her own journey—what would this do to mine and Julie's marriage?

It suddenly dawned on me that our lives had formed around the business of raising two kids. We'd done a great job, but now the heavy lifting was done. It was too late to get back to the way things used to be; that life had passed us by. I took a deep breath, went to a local flower shop, and bought a congratulatory bouquet. I was thrilled for Veronique, but now I knew that I would never return to the relationship that Julie and I had originally formed. Ultimately, I felt I was incapable of being the husband Julie needed and deserved.

Months turned into years as we stuck it out, but our lives remained distant. We tried seeing a marriage counselor, but it didn't help. During one session, while we explained our issues and the general emptiness we both felt, our counselor suddenly broke down in tears. In a moment that is certainly more humorous in retrospect than it was at the time, we found ourselves consoling the very person who was supposed to be helping us. I guess our story was just that sad (or the counselor was going through her own issues). Needless to say, the session finished rather awkwardly. When Julie and I went outside to the parking lot we looked at each other and wondered: "What do we do now?"

During this period I tended to work from home most days, and other than the occasional travel I was usually at my desk or in the living room. With the kids gone and nothing left to bind us together, I felt stressed when Julie got home—not because I didn't love her, but because the incompatibility that had lain under the surface was now staring me in the face. On the drive to visit Veronique and David we'd had serious conversations about what to do, but there was never a concluding statement or decision.

It was a long commute from Cantley to Julie's workplace on the other side of Ottawa. In late 2012 we agreed to buy a condo close to her work, partly as an investment and partly so she could avoid the long drive. Somehow that felt okay, until I mentioned the new arrangement at an appointment with my psychiatrist. He looked at me and expressed surprise that Julie and I were separated. At first I told him that we weren't separated, that it was just an arrangement for Julie's work. He looked at me again, this time staring into my eyes, and declared that Julie and I weren't living together, and that's what separated meant. Subconsciously, Julie and I had arranged our separation without even knowing it. We were no longer living alone together; we were now living alone under separate roofs.

In the spring of 2013 Julie officially moved out. I decided to get away to Cozumel, Mexico, for a week of scuba diving, in order to process the event and recalibrate my life. The thought of staying in the family home alone wasn't something I was prepared to deal with yet. While away I gathered my thoughts and tried to figure out what path to take next. When I got back to Cantley I decided to move to a cottage that we'd recently purchased and make it my new home. I spent the next seven months living alone. That summer I passed most days on the dock, staring at the island across the bay. The island seemed to represent how I'd experienced my life in recent years, as though I'd been living on an island, alone. But I enjoyed that summer nonetheless; it gave me time to think deeply about the various journeys I'd been on, and it enabled me to try to sort myself out.

By the early fall of 2013 Julie and I started to have some difficult conversations about what the future looked like. It became very clear to me from these discussions that my injury had really impacted her. And ironically, now that I was finally getting my feet under me again, it was Julie who was struggling. But since we couldn't figure out a way forward, our marriage continued to erode. In November, a woman whom I'd met during a business meeting approached me for a follow-up conversation. I responded by asking if she wanted to meet at her office or over a glass of wine. This was an unmistakable sign. When I drove home later that day I realized my marriage was over.

A few weeks later I visited Julie at her condo. She made us lunch, and when we sat down to eat I told her that I'd met someone. I'm not sure if I told her out of a desire to be honest, or simply to bring some conclusion after so much procrastinating about what we should do. She was stunned but very civil: I think she, too, knew that things were over. When lunch ended we hugged, cried for a few minutes, hugged again, and then I left. Our divorce became official in March 2014.

IN A TWIST of fate, when I returned from Afghanistan during the summer of 2007 Major-General Walter Semianiw was chief of military personnel. He'd been General Couture's chief of staff, and had called on me a few times to assist with high-profile issues related to how Canadian soldiers with mental health challenges were being treated, so he knew how effective the OSISS team was in supporting soldiers and their families. I felt that it was serendipitous that he was now in a position to further OSISS's cause and bring me back to the area I excelled at. Not long after I returned he got in touch and asked me to consider coming back to the military mental health world. Several months went by as we discussed what my role and mandate would be, which was trickier than it seemed, since he was essentially creating a position from scratch.

One day we met in his office. He said that he wanted to give me the title of "OSI special advisor." My main task would be to create and advance an educational program about OSIS that could be utilized throughout the entire Canadian Forces. General Semianiw understood that the next strategic step was to enhance the military's understanding of mental health in order to create widespread acceptance of OSIS and defeat prevalent stigmas. He was entrusting me with the duty to make that happen. That was a sizable challenge, since those in the clinical realm had traditionally been in charge of everything related to mental health. Soldiers didn't, and still don't, respond well to being lectured about the brain, so I knew we needed a new approach. Since officers were the ones in charge, they had to be made aware of mental health challenges; but equally important, we had to ensure that the rank and file understood and accepted them, too. Any changes had to come at the grassroots level as well, or else our efforts would be in vain.

After explaining what my role would be, General Semianiw looked me in the eye and calmly but sternly said, "This is not going to be an easy job. I will be loyal to you, but *do not fuck me.*" I must've looked quite surprised, because he immediately clarified himself: he knew there would be challenges, he explained, but under no circumstances did he want me going around him on an issue. This was a not-so-subtle reference to my email to Senator Dallaire in 2006 about the New Veterans Charter, which had caused some embarrassment to my previous boss, a vice admiral. Since I'd gone outside the chain of command before, General Semianiw wanted to make certain I wouldn't do the same to him.

I told him that he had my utmost loyalty, but that I also wanted to ensure I was protected. In a few years he would most likely be posted out to a higher position—something that often occurred with high-ranking officers—at which point someone else would step into his shoes, someone who may or may not care about soldiers' mental health. It might cost me my job if the next boss didn't see this issue as something worth their time and resources. At the end of our conversation, the general convinced me that he would make sure I was taken care of when the time came. I accepted his assurance in good faith, and we shook on it.

General Semianiw was a mover and shaker, and I had a lot of respect for him. Unlike most others in his position, he refused to just toe the party line. I got to witness this quality firsthand during one particular meeting with the surgeon general. I'd been asked my opinion on a certain issue to do with PTSD; I disagreed with what the majority of the room, including the surgeon general, had said, and stated as much. As I explained my case, she made a point of rolling her eyes, which General Semianiw caught as he scanned the room. He interrupted me, and in front of everyone asked her what was wrong, essentially challenging her to openly state her disagreement. I wanted to crawl under the table: as the highest-ranking person in the room he could get away with that, but I had to deal with these senior officers afterwards. When the meeting concluded I politely told him that I really appreciated his support, but asked that he refrain from putting me in those difficult positions, since the military medical system could make my life very difficult. General Semianiw agreed, and in the end he was true to his word and supported me whenever I needed him.

From 2007 to 2010 my job as OSI advisor to the military involved overseeing, to some degree, the peer support program, as well as rolling out an OSI education campaign within the forces. That work led to the development of the Road to Mental Readiness program, a pre-deployment program that tried to strengthen soldiers' ability to recognize mental health struggles while overseas, and which bolstered mental resilience by preparing them for various operational challenges.

At the same time the federal government was also taking steps to modernize mental health treatment across Canada. In 2007, the federal government created the Mental Health Commission of Canada (MHCC), a national non-profit organization tasked with improving the mental health system in Canada and changing public attitudes. The MHCC was created largely as a result of a 2006 Senate report on mental health in Canada titled "Out of the Shadows at Last." The report took a comprehensive look at federal "client groups" and highlighted the stigma, lack of funding, and turf wars that pervaded the Canadian mental health system. Among other things, the report showed how professional interests within the medical community ensured that self-help and peer support groups were underfunded, and that their voices were drowned out by doctors and other health professionals. The report was, and still is, a scathing indictment of how bureaucracy and territorialism negatively affect the very patients the health-care system is supposed to be helping. Funded by Health Canada and given a ten-year mandate (up to 2017), the MHCC was tasked with countering the problems highlighted by the senate committee and its fiery chairman, retired senator Michael Kirby.

Largely due to my experiences with the military health system, I was appointed to the MHCC's Workplace Advisory Committee in 2007. In that capacity I had multiple conversations about peer support and innovative ways of dealing with workplace mental health. Liaising with the MHCC made me realize there were numerous opportunities to widen the concept of peer support to include all Canadians. OSISS had pushed the military's awareness of mental health light years beyond where it had been, and I had dreams that a nationwide peer support program could achieve the same thing for civilians. I spoke with General Semianiw in the fall of 2009 (as predicted, he was about to be posted out to another position). During our chat I asked if he was still willing to help me, as per our agreement, and he replied in the affirmative.

I outlined for him my basic concept for a national peer support project. My goal was to create standards of practice and to move the yardstick for peer support well ahead of where it currently was. General Semianiw had been a strong supporter of OSISS, so this wasn't a tough sell. He said in no uncertain terms that if he received a request to second me to the MHCC he would accept it. I thanked him for honouring our informal deal, and immediately began putting together a small team to pitch my project to the commission. New avenues were beckoning.

Chapter 8

NEW ADVENTURES IN MENTAL HEALTH

A fter talking to General Semianiw I began planning my jump from military to civilian mental health projects. The MHCC's Workplace Advisory Committee was comprised of a body of volunteers that met regularly to—as the name suggests—discuss mental health in the workplace. On the committee I met, among others, Richard Dixon, the vice-president of human resources at Nav Canada; Mary Ann Baynton, a well-recognized consultant and expert in workplace mental health; and Ian Arnold, a widely respected retired surgeon and consultant in workplace health and safety who became the committee's chair in 2008. Ian, who'd worked with large companies, was a visionary guy. He commanded respect because of his vast knowledge and inclusive approach to health matters. The committee was full of smart and engaged people, and as I soon discovered, every time I mentioned the notion of peer support all eyes in the room lit up.

Technically the OSISS program was a workplace program, because the workplace—the military, under the DND and Veterans Affairs—paid for it. But the majority of the clients that OSISS served were not currently "in the workplace," since many had been released or retired. In this sense the program was a sort of hybrid—part workplace, part community-based initiative. Peer supporters working in the community dealt with a wide spectrum of people struggling with mental challenges. Although OSISS's clients mainly had OSIS, they experienced many of the hardships that community peer support workers saw: loss of employment, loss of shelter, lack of income and savings, no food in the fridge, etc. Those issues weren't normally encountered when operating a civilian workplace peer support program, because for the most part companies pay decent wages and employees in their programs don't often have the corollary issues listed above. Community peer support workers, on the other hand, dealt with all the by-products of mental illness. Put simply, veterans and their issues were closer in kind to community.

Veterans were encountering those same by-products of mental health issues, and with time I saw the similarities between what OSISS peer supporters faced and what community peer support programs were up against. Those connections led me to put forward something called the Peer Project. By that time I felt that peer support was the next best thing to, and a good adjunct for, clinical care, but that the existing peer support programs failed to articulate exactly what peer support accomplished, why it worked, and most importantly why the Canadian government should be investing more resources in it.

Since I was only on the MHCC's advisory committee, I, like the other members, had no say over the actual implementation of MHCC programs. But with a team of people that included Arnold, Baynton, and Dixon, I nonetheless helped develop an "unsolicited proposal." In the proposal, we articulated the thrust of our argument: an important piece was missing from the Canadian peer support field, something that could enlarge its presence and credibility; if certain aspects of peer support were strengthened, the concept could be embedded in the fabric of the health-care system, resulting in much better treatment outcomes. But governments and workplaces were focussed on clinical matters, since evidence-based medicine was, and still is, the easiest way for politicians, managers, and doctors to ensure they are crashed and all seven people were killed. Of course, casualties weren't an uncommon event in Afghanistan, but never in a hundred years did I think that they'd be soldiers who worked for me.

I spent the next hour trying to piece together exactly what had happened, but when I realized that I wouldn't be able to learn anything until the morning, I went for a walk across the sprawling Kandahar Airfield to clear my head. I was very disturbed, and I knew that my entire staff would be, too, when they got the news the next day. Priede's and Gilyeat's deaths caused a series of memories from Rwanda to flood back into my mind, some of which I hadn't thought about since the 1990s. It had been ten years, and I was in Afghanistan under very different circumstances, but all of the same feelings of guilt, anxiety, and loss arose inside of me and caused my mind to start spinning.

There was nothing I could have done to prevent my subordinates' deaths, but my moral compass nonetheless began flying all over the place. All of the could haves, would haves, and should haves in the world can't stop situations like that from getting to you, making you wonder if you are somehow responsible. The only thing I knew for sure was that two families were going to get phone calls that would change the course of their lives forever. Eventually, while walking past the base's various tents and buildings, I lost track of time, and I suddenly smelled the stench of sewage: in my fugue-like state I'd walked to the far end of the base and was now standing in front of the open-air sewage-treatment facilities. I did my best to collect my thoughts on the long walk back to my sleeping quarters.

While I sat in my office the next morning, still stunned by the previous night's events, a member of the forensic investigation team, a military police sergeant-major, came to see me. He introduced himself and told me that his job was to ensure that Corporal Priede's body was speedily and properly repatriated to his loved ones. When he spoke I could tell from his beleaguered tone of voice that he'd been forced to perform this grim task numerous times already. He also added that, thankfully, Priede, Gilyeat, and the others died quickly and probably didn't feel anything. It was a small bit of consolation, but I was gutted nonetheless.

After the shock subsided, my thoughts immediately drifted to Corporal Priede's family in Canada. When I left for Afghanistan the OSISS HOPE program had been in full swing. Once I knew that Corporal Priede's family had received the tragic news I sent a message to the OSISS team to ensure that they didn't forget to offer their services. Sadly, I was now calling upon the very program I'd helped launch to aid a fallen comrade's family.

Years later Corporal Priede's mother Roxanne became a volunteer for the HOPE bereavement program, and in 2012 she attended the Remembrance Day ceremonies in Ottawa as a Silver Cross Mother. I made sure to meet with her and her husband John during one of their visits to Ottawa, to answer any questions they had about Darrell's death and give them my condolences. One small bit of comfort I got from that sad chapter was the knowledge that at least the program I created was helping the Priede family, who in turn were helping others in similar circumstances.

DAYS WERE LONG in Afghanistan. Most of the time I woke up early in the morning, worked until ten or eleven at night, crashed, and woke up to do it all again the following day. When I needed to decompress I lay on my cot, turned on my iPod, and did some Sudoku puzzles until I was tired. While going through that routine I often found my mind drifting off, to thoughts of a more enjoyable home life after Afghanistan. I kept thinking, hoping: "Things are going to be better when I get back."

Deploying to Rwanda in 1994 changed the dynamic of family life in my house. To be sure, the kids grew up to be just fine—they were everything we could've hoped for—but over the years my marriage slowly eroded. Julie and I still loved one another, but we weren't *in love* anymore. Our household ran smoothly enough, but we both spent most of our time alone. As the saying goes, we were strangers under the same roof. I'll never know for certain if my marriage would've eroded regardless of my time in Rwanda, but the difficulties I faced afterward definitely drove a wedge between us, one that we getting the most bang for their buck. They were hesitant to try any new methods unless those methods had a pile of studies supporting their effectiveness. For that reason we knew we had an uphill battle ahead of us.

The Peer Project was based on two of my beliefs. The first was that we needed more true *peers*—those who know what it's like to live with mental health challenges—in peer support roles. In order to achieve that goal, we needed to create the conditions for peer support to receive funding. This was connected to my second belief: that clear standards of practice had to be developed and implemented. Once standards were created, peer support could be precisely defined, as opposed to letting it be defined by anyone who said "I'm a peer supporter." Clearly defined standards meant the concept of peer support would be enhanced in the eyes of physicians, that politicians and administrators would be willing to devote resources to it, and that everyone could see what they were getting for their money. We knew our position would isolate a certain percentage of existing peer supporters and programs—those who favoured a very informal approach—but strategic change always makes some people uncomfortable. I for one thought the changes were worthwhile.

Another component of the Peer Project was the notion that in our quest to de-stigmatize mental illness and enhance mental health literacy in Canada, peers—people who have experienced mental health challenges—should be leveraged to help others. Unbeknownst to me, the MHCC already had its own initiative to combat stigma, so that aspect of our proposal was considered redundant to their needs.

The MHCC had commissioned its own study, called "Making the Case for Peer Support," which was released in September 2010. Unfortunately, I think most people who took the time to read it would look up afterward and think, "They didn't make the case." Indeed, it failed to lay the grounds for furthering peer support because it didn't outline any changes that would strategically alter clinical and governmental perspectives. I don't want to denigrate the enormous amount of work that went into it—including the creation of focus groups and consultations with several hundred patients, practitioners, and policy-makers—but, concisely put, the report was very anecdotal and it didn't express any tangible ways to change the system. It affirmed (or rather re-affirmed) that peer support worked, that there was a growing evidence base to support the practice, and that the clinical approach was only part of the mental health solution. Basically, the report concluded by saying that the MHCC needed to work to change the system with those who'd experienced mental health challenges, and that the new system had to be inclusive—a vague conclusion, to say the least.

Ultimately it was still just a report, and oftentimes reports that lack any strong conclusions fail to translate into tangible action. In fact, most often in the twenty-first century, reports seem to just lead to further studies and reports. But while the MHCC, based on its original mandate, couldn't deliver actual services, it did have a transformational leadership role to play. I welcomed this, because the Peer Project my colleagues and I put together aimed to go beyond the more limited vision outlined in the commission's report. We wanted the MHCC to be an incubator, over a five-year period, for a new organization that could grow out of the commission, something that could provide both certification and accreditation services for peer support in Canada, and conduct further research into peer support's value. That would be something *tangible*, something that could further drive the implementation and standardization of peer support across the country and help to legitimize it in the eyes of medical professionals, politicians, and the public.

With the support of the Workplace Advisory Committee and the MHCC's vice president of research, Dr. Jayne Barker, our proposal was submitted to the commission's board of directors at their 2010 meeting in Saskatoon. The response from the board was positive, and very quickly the commission said it wanted in on the action. Shortly after that, Senator Kirby wrote a letter to the military asking that I be seconded to the commission. The timing worked perfectly, since General Semianiw's new posting was now proceeding and his departure was imminent. He could then make good on his word, ensuring that I was taken care of as we'd agreed. He accepted my secondment, and the next thing I knew I was starting what I thought would be a five-year journey with the MHCC to create the Peer Project.

I STARTED AT the commission in April 2010. Like kids do on the first day of school, I tried to ingratiate myself to everyone at the commission's Ottawa office. Though I maintained my office at the DND, and was still available to General Semianiw, I tried to get to know other commission members whenever I could.

Unfortunately, after talking with several I came to the conclusion that many of them meant well but liked to grandstand and lacked substance. They knew all the buzzwords, fashionable terms like *patient-centred care*, and they spoke a lot about the need to decrease stigma, but there wasn't much behind what they said. Most of what they discussed was purely academic, and coming from a position where I'd dealt with workplace mental health firsthand, a lot of their words struck me as just more of the same talk that always led to more studies and little action. I was looking for people with insight, vision, and the energy to get things done. I looked forward to learning from the other commission members, but sadly, after several months of liaising and talking with them I realized that, with a few notable exceptions, they didn't have any big plans. That was a scary thought, since they were at the Mental Health Commission of Canada, an organization tasked with changing our approach to mental health.

The first time I spoke on the phone with a senior individual (also a volunteer with the MHCC) at a local branch of the Canadian Mental Health Association in Toronto, I could tell he loved to hear the sound of his own voice. Without exaggeration, my cell phone ran out of battery life before he ran out of breath. Almost his entire monologue was about how many contacts he had and how much he knew; the rest of the time he patronizingly explained that, since I was from the military, I had no idea how community mental health worked. He was correct that I had a lot to learn about community mental health, but he was wrong in thinking that there was no need to further advance the function of peer support. Nonetheless, he essentially told me that since the commission had already published "Making the Case for Peer Support," its work was done. He then went on to list the names of people who would be against my project. From our conversation I gathered that he was a glass-is-half-empty kind of guy, and that if an idea wasn't his, it was a bad one.

He was half right that some people, like Diana Capponi, a tireless advocate for the mentally ill who passed away in 2014, would *initially* be against my ideas. Diana had an amazing and inspiring story. She was a survivor of sexual abuse and heroin addiction, and later worked at Toronto's Centre for Addiction and Mental Health, ensuring that both past and present patients were provided paid employment there when opportunities arose. She of all people knew what mental illness looked like and how complex the issue was. When I met with her she was worried about marginalizing peer supporters, overcomplicating things, and potentially closing the door to peers without higher education who might nonetheless be great at helping others. These were all legitimate concerns. But she kept an open mind, and in the time it took us to enjoy a coffee together, she became interested in my ideas; she felt that, with the proper chiseling, they could work.

As it so happened, Diana later became a board director at Peer Support Accreditation and Certification Canada, which I helped found, where she was instrumental in helping create a rigorous but grounded process for peer support accreditation. Simply put, she was nothing like the Diana that had been described to me, and I quickly learned that myopic thinking was rampant among some people in the mental health field, including at the commission. There were some great individuals associated with the MHCC, especially those I worked with on the advisory committee, but it was also clear that a lot of people charged with changing the system in Canada were the ones partially responsible for the system's shortfalls in the first place.

While creating the peer support standards of practice I collaborated with Dr. Rachel Thibault, a pioneer in community-based rehabilitation. I'd met Rachel several years earlier when she accompanied some of her University of Ottawa students as they interviewed me about my work at the DND. I knew that her fount of knowledge would be instrumental as I moved forward. Supported by the MHCC, Rachel and I travelled the country, meeting with a multitude of peer supporters who worked in the medical system or with community services. She brought scientific rigour and a disciplined approach that complemented my rather informal tactics.

One factor that made the project to create peer support standards more difficult—and that once again spoke to the rampant territorialism among some health-care professionals—was the stonewalling I received when trying to gather the names of existing peer supporters. When we started compiling a list of these individuals, the MHCC's "Making the Case" report had already helped create a massive database of several hundred peer supporters across the country. But even though I was working under the MHCC's auspices, when I tried to get access to this database I was subjected to delays, bogus confidentiality excuses, and even denials.

Eventually I changed my approach and explored how to create our own database. Mary Ann Baynton offered the help of her son Spencer, and two of Spencer's friends, David MacDonald and Brandon Mirrlees, who were familiar with computer software and other technical aspects I didn't know the first thing about. Together they (voluntarily) spent countless hours doing Google searches and using other strategies to compile a database of over six hundred people in the peer support field across Canada. Ultimately, their efforts helped us to separate our project from the MHCC's earlier initiative, therefore avoiding some of its members' territorial posturing.

After contacting peer supporters we set up day-long qualitative research consultations with Dr. Thibault, still thankfully supported by Dr. Jayne Barker and the MHCC. These sessions took place in Halifax, Quebec City, Montreal, Toronto, Ottawa, Calgary, and Vancouver, and they included a few hundred people from our database who'd agreed to meet with us. Each consultation had anywhere from fifteen to thirty-five people. Rachel or I usually opened the conversation by explaining our intention to create standards of practice for peer support in Canada. We then spent the rest of the day talking with them about all aspects of the subject, including things like competencies and codes of conduct. Our main goal was to understand what skills, abilities, and knowledge were crucial for peer supporters. Once these sessions were complete we organized the data as best we could and then handed our work over to another volunteer, Annette Ducharme, who tried to fit what we'd learned into various conceptual categories, out of which we fashioned a peer support framework.

When this process was complete the final results were put into an online survey. Participants were then invited to give us their thoughts about every aspect of the framework. Afterwards we sent a note to all six hundred people in our database asking them to provide us with the names of those knowledgeable in the subject who they felt best represented their views. The names that appeared the most were made part of a peer leaders group. These people helped us to refine our standards of practice by discussing peer support, coming up with ways to promote it, and deciding what guidelines should govern its use. Wendy Mishkin, who was with the Victoria branch of the British Columbia Schizophrenia Society, helped us compile everything into a complex knowledge matrix that we used to establish knowledge and performance targets, so that organizations that wanted to professionalize their peer support program could rigorously audit how they trained peer supporters. Kim Sunderland was another crucial contributor; she worked to develop "Standards of Practice for Peer Support," a report that outlined the qualifications necessary for peer support certification.

This was supposed to be a five-year project, and by accepting it the MHCC had agreed to be an incubator for an organization that would oversee the accreditation process for peer support in Canada. Unfortunately, institutional turmoil and personal machinations at the MHCC partially derailed us after less than two years of effort. In 2012 my boss on the project, Dr. Jayne Barker, was effectively fired by the MHCC's president (her contract was not renewed). As a senior vice-president at the commission she was a force to be reckoned with,* and from the

---

*   Jayne was also the key person in the "Homeless Project" conducted under the MHCC's auspices.

very first she saw the long-term strategic value of furthering peer support. Although I can't say for sure, I believe that sticking her neck out for us was one of the reasons her contract wasn't renewed.

After Jayne's departure the project struggled. Without her leadership and clout we were marginalized within the MHCC. We tried to impress upon the commission's senior executives the value of our work for *all* Canadians, but over time it became obvious that they were finished with us. Eventually, our budget was slashed and the project was cancelled. I felt terrible. I had put all my trust in the commission, had met with hundreds of Canadians dedicated to peer support, and had stuck my own neck out when I told people that we must work together and that the MHCC would support us. I felt like I'd let them all down. But after witnessing firsthand how powerful peer support had been for numerous men and women in the military, I couldn't fathom simply letting the project go.

With important work left to do, Rachel, Ian Arnold, and I decided to go ahead without the MHCC. When I surveyed the Canadian peer support field, it quickly became evident that it was divided into roughly two camps. On one side there was the "consumer-survivors," usually former patients of the mental health system who'd literally *survived* it, despite the system's perceived wrongdoings. They were great people, but a lot of them had a very polarized and negative view of the medical system, and most were not amenable to working within the system in order to change it: a lot of them viewed doctors as the enemy, and they wished to keep anyone with a formal education out of peer support. On the other side were social workers—some of whom had lived with a mental illness themselves. Many of these individuals had participated in ACT (assertive community treatment) teams, helping mentally ill patients in their daily lives. They did great work, but my problem with this form of peer support was that, as strange as it might sound, some people can be overqualified for peer support.

To clarify: someone still on their journey to recovery will, for the most part, be more likely to empathize with a peer dealing with mental health problems, since their own struggles are still fresh in their mind. In some cases, time and distance can make it more difficult for the recovered to empathize with the still-recovering. Formal education, too, as important as it is in many areas of medical care, can breed a sense of objectivity that is at odds with human nature. For a surgeon who needs to operate on a diseased organ, the ability to coldly and methodically work without emotion is crucial. But for a peer supporter, it is important to constantly be connected to their peer's journey (within reason, of course). The ability to remember how it feels to have a drug problem, to live on the streets, or to feel scared to leave the house is essential. Formal education, combined with time and distance, can sometimes engender a completely detached approach to mental health problems. That, in my estimation, is not peer support.

Meeting different types of peer supporters across Canada was crucial because it allowed me to see the entire spectrum of peer support, and to understand how each group approached the subject. Those meetings also allowed me to witness how peer support could be twisted for ulterior purposes.

One telling anecdote involved a meeting with the director of a homeless shelter. I'd been told that it was essential to meet with this person, I suspect because she intended to show me how "real" peer support was done. When I arrived the woman was at first polite and hospitable, but she nonetheless seemed hostile to my project. She was, like many individuals in the field, worried that professionalizing peer support would lead to it being overtaken by the medical system, rather than the two systems working alongside each other. She took me on a tour of the shelter, and at one point introduced me to a dishwasher, who was also apparently a peer supporter. As it turned out, part of the shelter's provincial funding went to "peer support," which the director then used for running the shelter—in this case, to pay a dishwasher. As far as I could gather, he was a peer supporter in title only, and did no actual peer support. I understood the director's desire to obtain funding however she could, and of course she had to employ a dishwasher. But leveraging peer support funding in that way made me uncomfortable. This may have been a pragmatic attempt to ensure the shelter's survival, but I was still disheartened to see peer support used in a manner other than its intended purpose.

My tour of the homeless shelter taught me a lot about why government officials and clinicians were always slightly reserved about peer support. Any politician or doctor visiting that shelter who knew nothing about the subject would've been similarly confused: "This guy doing the dishes is a peer supporter?" That example was, in my mind, one of the reasons why peer support was rarely taken seriously.

This reminded me of a meeting I had in the winter of 2011 with peer supporters from across Canada. Halfway through, a woman stood up and said she was sick of all the talk about re-engineering peer support. She couldn't understand why governments and medical professionals didn't just *trust* that peer supporters knew what they were doing. As she finished talking a smirk came across her face; it seemed to dawn on her that, given the many types of "peer support" across Canada, the answer was obvious. Indeed, there was no common understanding of what constitutes peer support—a problem that left funding bodies justifiably puzzled about what taxpayers' money was being used for. Gaining the co-operation and support of governments and clinicians meant standardizing peer support qualifications, laying out specific guidelines about what peer support entailed, and demonstrating that it wasn't just an amorphous idea with a thousand different meanings. There was so much passion and effort by peer supporters everywhere, but the field was chaotic and uncoordinated.

My colleagues on the Peer Project and I tried to convince skeptics that harnessing all of that energy and effort could produce wonders. Our group wanted to produce a standard form of peer support that wouldn't be co-opted by "the system" but would nonetheless be rigorous and accountable—two qualities sorely missing from the current plethora of peer supports out there. Many of the well-meaning individuals practicing what they felt was the best type of peer support wanted funding but were unwilling to be accountable to their funders. They essentially wanted the system to contribute to their cause, but didn't want the system to ask any questions about what they were doing, or whether what they were doing actually worked.

That was just plain naive. We could all agree that the end goal was to make life easier for those suffering with mental health challenges, so it made no sense to fragment ourselves instead of working together. Fears of big government and bureaucracy, or being lost in the system, needed to be replaced with a belief that the team approach was better than everyone working in their own corner. Our goal wasn't to produce bean counters or peer supporters who would check their watch every few minutes to see if the scheduled meeting time was up. We weren't the enemy, nor did we unabashedly kowtow to the system. But it took time to convince people of that.

Eventually, when the Peer Project was terminated in early 2012 there was a drawn-out discussion about the intellectual property of the material we'd developed. I was under a secondment from the DND, and the project was conducted under the MHCC's auspices, so it was logical that they wanted to keep it for themselves. But based on past experience I was concerned that it would not lead to any specific, tangible improvements. But thanks to the creative thinking of Sapna Mahajan, a trusted employee of the MHCC, Kim Sunderland was hired to use the material to create both general and training guidelines for peer support. Both were subsequently published by the MHCC. This meant that all of the knowledge we'd gained from the project was translated into another report that would be available to all Canadians, thereby ensuring that it could be used to drive further improvements in peer support.

The MHCC had to justify to its funder, Health Canada, all the work we'd conducted, and even though we'd produced yet another report, it was a solid one. When our separation from the MHCC occurred we were able to retain the standards of practice and use them to develop the "Credentialing Process for Peer Support" report, while the MHCC saved face and published their guidelines, which were based on the same knowledge and data from our work over the past two years.

GIVEN THAT WE saw the break from the MHCC coming, in 2011 Ian Arnold, Rachel Thibault, and I decided to pre-emptively start the process of incorporating a new, non-profit charity for our work: Peer Support Accreditation and Certification (Canada) (PSACC).

I was happy to carry on such important work, but I also felt like it was ridiculous that three Canadian citizens had to shoulder the burden of making it happen with literally nothing—no funding or initial support. Creating a non-profit organization is quite a daunting task, but thankfully Ian, with the assistance of Ted Ormston (chair of the MHCC's Law Advisory Committee), was able to find us some pro bono legal assistance to sort out the labyrinthine paperwork and get things moving. By this point, my marriage was falling apart, and I'd decided to retire from the military after twenty-nine years, so needless to say, I didn't have much time to dedicate to the endeavour. And so the burden was on Ian's and Rachel's shoulders as they worked to get PSACC off the ground.

After PSACC was legally incorporated in late 2011, we hired Kim Sunderland to be our executive director. Our task was clear: we had to take all of the research we'd accumulated and devise a certification process and testing methods for peer support. Minutiae such as record keeping and ensuring people abided by a code of conduct were crucial for guaranteeing that peer support worked and was respected by professionals and policy-makers. Equally important was the creation of a nationwide cadre of mentors who were capable of training peer supporters in both clinical and community mental health settings.

Fortuitously, in the spring of 2012 the province of Nova Scotia unveiled its Mental Health and Addictions Strategy, which aimed at, among other things, health promotion, early intervention in mental health crises, and closing gaps in the current system. I met several provincial representatives during my time with the MHCC, and they were quite interested in the peer support credentialing process. That interest led to the province becoming essentially our first "client." On the heels of PSACC's creation we obtained a contract with Nova Scotia to increase the presence and prominence of peer support in its provincial mental health system. The credentialing process was instrumental in providing clinicians with a solid understanding of what peer supporters brought to the table, and it demonstrated the rigour we would bring to peer support.

PSACC's contract with the government of Nova Scotia gave us the kick-start we required, and it provided the organization with some much-needed cachet. PSACC (of which I am president) continues to grow, with the tripartite mission of promoting the recognition, growth, and accessibility of peer support for all Canadians. That mission is achieved above all by using the aforementioned standards of practice to promote mental health support through education and awareness, certifying qualified peer supporters, and accrediting qualified peer support training programs. All of this is done using rigorous research methodologies that are expanding the evidence base for peer support and demonstrating its effectiveness. I saw the immense value of peer support for military members and veterans, and now I'm slowly starting to witness the same effect in the civilian realm. That progress makes all of the setbacks and hardship worth it.

DURING MY TIME working with the MHCC I was invited on numerous occasions to discuss the Peer Project at conferences and other venues in the Canadian mental health field. This allowed me to connect with businesses and their human-resources staff, as well as with a plethora of people working in mental health across Canada.

The story was always the same with respect to how companies dealt with mental health: disability-management workers managing disabilities when it was too late; cookie-cutter (and often inadequately resourced) employee-assistance programs; insurance companies handling the financial side of things, sometimes with little care for anything else; and performance-management staff conducting— no surprise—performance management, with very little idea of how to deal with their employees' underlying issues. In short, there was a lot of room for improvement.

I knew that if we were going to tackle the mental health problem, people had to start thinking outside the box. Canadians cannot keep relying solely on governments to provide mental health solutions: employers should share some responsibility for fixing this problem as well. After learning about the mental health field I became convinced

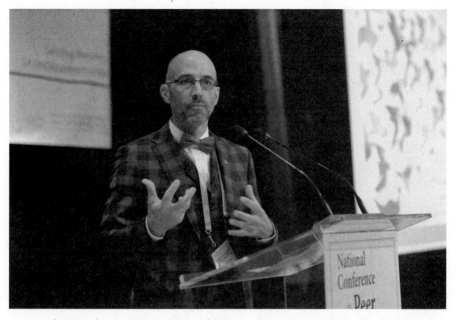

Speaking at the 2016 National Conference on Peer Support, Toronto, Ontario. Photo: Andre Apperley.

that Canadian workplaces needed to step up and not just donate to charitable organizations through their corporate responsibility programs, but also provide their employees with tangible help. Despite the satisfaction I got from working with other volunteers to achieve PSACC's objectives, in my personal life I had only half a pension from the military (the rest went to Julie), and I needed to devise other ways to make a living. I also had to find ways to obtain funding for the new charity, a task that over time would prove very difficult. And so my accountant convinced me to create a small business as a means to bill for conference presentations and provide funding for day-to-day activities. Slowly, I began to put together Mental Health Innovations (MHI).

I started with just one contract with NAV Canada, a not-for-profit corporation that owns and operates Canada's civil air navigations system; I was tasked with helping them to implement their own peer support program. The aviation industry is a very stressful one. I'd met with NAV's vice-president of human resources when I was a member of the MHCC's Workforce Advisory Committee, and the concept of peer support resonated with him. And when I met with Lyne Wilson, NAV's human resources director, she immediately understood the benefits of such a program. Like others who'd witnessed the power of peer support firsthand, the people at NAV became champions of the concept, and theirs was one of the first organizations to begin reshaping how Canadian corporations handle mental health.

When researching what other Canadian corporations and governments were doing for employees with mental health problems, it seemed to me that a lot of organizations were abdicating their responsibilities in this area; indeed, many seemed concerned more with image than changing the status quo. Some gave millions to charity but left their own employees out in the cold.

One company—it shall remain nameless—was a particularly egregious example of this contradictory stance. Employees I met were unanimous in stating that while their managers were not bad people, the dominant corporate culture prevented anyone from truly supporting those with mental health problems. On several occasions, employees stayed behind after the official meetings we had with their company, and they often broke down when asking us for advice. One woman explained how she was distraught because she suffered from severe bleeding during her menses: she had been scolded by her manager for her frequent (short) absences while she attended to her needs. Understandably, she felt embarrassed and demeaned at having to explain the situation. Other employees told me about the constant feeling of being at the mercy of the clock, since the company kept track of their work *to the minute*, chastising them for the slightest infraction. To some degree I couldn't help but be reminded of my military days when hearing these stories. The essential attitude was, "suck it up or get out and find a job elsewhere."

If a company doesn't care about its employees' mental health and gives no money to charity, they aren't acting respectably, but at least they're being honest. In my opinion, it's worse to donate money to various causes but then simultaneously indicate to your employees that you don't care about mental health in your own backyard. I've always said that mental illness is like bad breath—you don't smell your own; you only smell it on others. For some companies it was and still is just about public image.

THERE ARE OBVIOUS differences between physical and mental injuries. For example, if I break my leg, my belief in my body's natural ability to heal has very little to do with the healing process; so long as I comply with the treatment, the physiological processes will continue, regardless of my thoughts about it. Society, however, often makes two big mistakes about mental health. The first is underestimating and undervaluing the input of the mentally injured. We usually assume that they're too fragile, or that their opinions are flawed because of their mental state. The second is underestimating the important role that *belief* in recovery can play. Unlike a broken leg, believing that I can heal my broken mind helps my healing process. That is where peer support comes in. Peer support provides someone in the abyss of despair a tangible example that someone else was once in a similar position, and they nonetheless recovered. For the ill person, their peer becomes living proof that they, too, can look forward to better days. Once that connection is made, the journey to recovery is helped immensely. The same phenomenon is often seen in cancer survivors.

What society needs to do is stop *talking* about the one-in-five who suffer from mental illness, and start *engaging* with them. No matter what conference you attend on mental health in Canada, within the first hour you'll hear that one-in-five Canadians suffers from a mental health problem, and that it costs Canadian society $50 billion or more per year—and that the cost is still rising. My philosophy—and one that I try to impart to people wherever I go—is simple: let's stop talking *about* those who need help and start talking *with* them. One of the pillars of future success will be making those with mental health challenges part of the solution, and this will only happen when organizations create meaningful peer support programs.

The initial corporate reaction to this idea is usually something like this: "You don't understand, there's so much stigma, no one is ever going to come to the meeting or be seen coming to the meeting." But I can tell you from firsthand experience with members of the military, perhaps the most reticent of all Canadians to discuss their mental health problems: it's all in the presentation. If you write a memo that says, "We are looking to improve mental health outcomes, and so we've hired an expert team that wants to meet any employee who has suffered from a mental illness," then of course no one is going to show up—stigmas about mental illness are still too strong. On the other hand, if the memo says something like, "The experts we've hired want to consult our employees and obtain input about how the company can better support staff dealing with mental health problems," people are less worried about coming because you haven't singled out the participants as necessarily having a mental health problem themselves.

Anecdotally, we know that those who come to these types of meetings are aware of what we're talking about and are willing to work overtime that day to ensure they can attend, because they value the fact that the company is doing something to make things better. They really want to share their opinions, and they really want to see changes. For the company, this strategy allows managers to achieve their objective without violating their employees' confidentiality. In my experience, such meetings have also been well attended by caring and interested employees without mental health problems, since they, too, want to see their colleagues happy.

Engaging people who've lived through a mental health problem helps achieve important goals. Namely, it provides helpful insight into the company's organizational culture. Unfortunately, employees often feel that the company they work for is itself part of the problem, and many times they are correct. By learning what they can do better, companies can positively change organizational culture and make their employees' work lives easier. That is especially crucial for those dealing with mental health challenges.

WHEN CANADIANS ARE mentally unwell at work, usually the only tangible things they are offered are an employee assistance program (EAP) or a clinical intervention. That is not enough. We need complementary programs to ensure people recover properly.

It's often not until an employee has a crisis at work that employers recognize there is any kind of issue. And even when companies do recognize that there is an issue, how are managers trained to deal with it? They bring the person into their office, conduct a performance appraisal, possibly (and often subtly) refer them to the EAP, and if they're an experienced and empathetic manager, have a closed-door, heart-to-heart discussion. While those steps are helpful, they can't always ensure success. A manager can be very adroit when dealing with an employee in trouble or in recovery, but that journey can take a year or longer, and if the manager is the only person providing support, that simply isn't sufficient. What's more, all of this assumes that the manager is a skilled and compassionate person. Sadly, in a lot of cases managers are great at performance managing but provide very little moral support. That can make the situation even worse for someone facing mental health challenges.

In addition, if you look at the situation from the employee's perspective, they don't want to knock on their manager's door every other day for a twenty-minute conversation. They may feel it is inappropriate. They know that their manager isn't paid to have heart-to-hearts, and very quickly they feel uncomfortable with approaching their boss every time they feel the need to speak with someone. Simply put, managers can't do it all.

The workplace model for dealing with health matters is heavily skewed towards physical injuries; it is very predictive and prescriptive: you broke your leg, you are going to need some time to recover, and then you'll be back to work. EAPs, which trace their beginnings in Canada to the 1940s, stem largely from occupational alcoholism treatment programs, which aimed to help employees during a time when drinking (and being drunk) on the job was relatively common. Like most programs, they evolved over time.

EAPs were and are important for employees' health and productivity, but they've also have proved ineffective against the tsunami of mental health challenges that twenty-first-century workplaces face. Many EAPs cover six to eight therapy sessions, and no more, essentially cutting things off right when the person is starting to make headway. Even if the provincial health-care system takes over afterward, that still means starting the journey over again with a different therapist. Care in the Canadian mental health system can sometimes be very disjointed, and often the EAP structure compounds that problem.

With these challenges in mind, it's easy to see how a peer support program can help plug these gaps and provide a non-clinical form of support that reflects the hectic and fragmented nature of twenty-first-century employment and life.

ONE OF THE points I always stress when talking about mental health is that we currently don't engage people in the "seven-to-ten" zone. Draw in your mind a vertical line with zero at the bottom and ten at the top. Zero represents the completely stress-free person (if that's even possible), while ten would be someone who is suicidal. Rare are the human beings that live entirely at zero or ten. We go through all sorts of ups and downs in our lifetime, and most of us tend to slide up and down the scale depending on what's happening in our lives.

Let me give a few personal examples. After my son was born, like most new parents I didn't sleep much; this put me at around a three on the zero-to-ten scale. This minor disruption to my normal rhythm was an accepted part of being a new parent, and it was something that I openly discussed with other men in my regiment. But later in life, when I was experiencing the mental fallout of Rwanda, I was often living in the seven or eight zone, and though it was obvious to those around me that I was unwell, no one wanted to engage me. When my father passed away, by contrast, I was somewhere around a four or a five. I was obviously upset and grieving, but since his passing was expected and life was otherwise going well, I was able to cope.

The difference between these three examples is that, both socially and at work, people are willing to engage those in the one-to-six zone, whereas they aren't willing to engage those in the seven-to-ten zone. We are taught by society that unless speaking with close friends or family, the seven-to-ten zone is awkward and taboo. If people see that I'm at a nine and am about to blow my top, no one wants to approach and say, "Hey, Stéphane, are you doing okay?" Only family and very close friends will do that. But if I spend most of my day at work, what do I do when I'm feeling miserable for those eight hours, hours that gradually add up to weeks and months?

On the other hand, the example of my father's passing demonstrates that when people are in the one-to-six zone, colleagues are quite happy to offer condolences and go through all of the social niceties we are trained to deploy under such circumstances. When a person is in that comfortable range we will engage with them; when they're beyond that point, we shy away. What we need is a breakthrough, a change of attitude, and most importantly a new approach. When people are in that uncomfortable seven-to-ten zone, the zone we are least willing to engage with, that is when they need others the most. Once again, I believe that peer support can help bridge that gap and make a difference, the way it made a difference in my life and the lives of thousands of others over the past decade.

Conclusion

PRESCRIPTIONS FOR CHANGE

I n the late 1990s the Canadian military was just beginning to discuss mental trauma. Outside of medical circles, Canadians had little understanding at the time of what PTSD was. But in the two decades since, though Canadians have become interested in mental trauma and PTSD, the pendulum has swung too fast and too far in the opposite direction. We now rarely go a single week without seeing trauma or PTSD discussed in national newspapers or on television: trauma and PTSD are everywhere.

For example, several provinces—at the time of this writing, Alberta, Saskatchewan, Manitoba, and Ontario—have recently enacted PTSD legislation for emergency first responders, which has established the disorder as a presumptive occupational illness. On the face of it, such legislation is a welcome development. Recognizing and accepting that there are significant mental health risks for those in difficult jobs is a long-overdue step in the right direction, especially because it signifies that we're beginning to treat mental and physical health with equal respect. Unfortunately, this legislation could potentially create some unintended consequences.

During my time working on mental health in the military, I coined the term *operational stress injury*, in part for soldiers who were morally unwell but did not necessarily have PTSD. The unintended consequence of drawing so much attention to PTSD was that many troops felt they had it, when in fact they had depression (which was more common) or another mental health issue. With the OSI concept I attempted to steer military culture away from presupposing a PTSD diagnosis, because this also predetermined soldiers' care and treatment. Unfortunately, I was only somewhat successful. Over time, PTSD became the default, catch-all diagnosis for military members. And now, it seems, PTSD has become the go-to diagnosis for first responders and many others, too.

I've heard directly from first responders that well-intentioned colleagues sometimes now encourage them to "get" a PTSD diagnosis and seek medical care for any occupational incident. In addition, some in the legal industry have caught on to the rise of PTSD diagnoses and use it for their own gain. Unscrupulous lawyers specializing in car accident cases find equally unscrupulous doctors to provide their client with a PTSD diagnosis, even if the accident was the most minor of fender-benders.

The public has gotten caught up in this PTSD frenzy, too. Several doctors have related to me how distraught patients now often arrive at their office with the predetermined notion that they have PTSD. We have reached the point where PTSD is threatening to become the diagnosis de jour for almost everyone who suffers any form of emotional hardship, however minor. These are dangerous waters to swim in.

PTSD has become somewhat of a Canadian national obsession. One need only pick up any major newspaper, like the *Toronto Star* or the *Globe and Mail*, to see how preoccupied we've become with both trauma and PTSD. Every week, it seems, there are multiple articles about PTSD among first responders, members of the military, journalists, and now even health-care workers themselves. In July 2016, the *Guardian*, a leading British newspaper, examined the findings of an academic study that reported that not only are PTSD rates higher in affluent countries—Canada ranks highest among them.

According to the study, those who are accustomed to tough living but who lack complex medical services are, paradoxically, *less* likely to develop PTSD than those living in relative luxury with access to a rigorous health-care system. While some of this may be explained by the lack of medical services in impoverished countries—which may preclude any PTSD diagnoses in the first place (no psychiatrists, no diagnoses)—it may also reflect the possibility that in our rush to find trauma everywhere we may be unintentionally convincing many that they have PTSD when their malady is something different, perhaps something in the moral or spiritual realm. Chris Brewin from University College London, a leading trauma researcher and a co-author of the study, has argued that if we are brought up to believe that the world is a safe place and people mean well toward us, our mind is much more likely to be traumatized when we discover otherwise. On the other hand, those from poor countries, who are used to dealing with danger and adversity, are not as surprised when something traumatic or evil occurs.

What is going on here? Unfortunately, as is often the case with scientific research, Brewin and his colleagues concluded that more work needs to be done. As Canadians, though, at the very least this study should cause us to reflect on whether our trauma obsession has gone too far.

Despite being diagnosed with PTSD myself, I believe our fixation on trauma has become at best unhelpful, and at worst dangerous. We have gradually developed a psychiatric system whose very rigid diagnostic processes are in many cases funneling people into a PTSD diagnosis, when they may in fact be dealing with other mental issues. As we continue to explore the various conditions that people develop in the workplace—whether they're police, paramedics, soldiers, or anyone that is subjected to significant hardship or trauma—I would argue that the concepts of stress and moral injuries need to be further examined. There are multiple causes behind mental deterioration—trauma, grief, fatigue, and moral conflict being prevalent among them. With regard to trauma—or grief, which can be traumatic in its own right—it is easy to see how someone can develop PTSD; but what about the other two? I'm not convinced that someone who has worked extremely hard or gone through significant moral conflict should be told they have PTSD.

So much attention has been given to the concept of trauma that we're at the point where people with hurt feelings claim they are traumatized. In my work with the Canadian public, I've been told things like, "my boss's email traumatized me," and "I was traumatized when my manager said my position may be eliminated next year."

The unintended effect is that Canadians are now coming to their own conclusions about what constitutes trauma. Unfortunately, this trend is only exacerbated by modern technology. The Internet allows anyone to conduct their own mental health research. People go online, read about symptoms, connect the dots, and then make the conclusion that they have PTSD. More often than not, they are incorrect. Statistically, depression, which was a cultural obsession in the 1980s and '90s, is more common than PTSD, yet PTSD is invoked to a much higher degree. While I can only guess at what is driving this trend—the medicalization of everyday life perhaps—I can nonetheless state with certainty that our obsession with trauma can do serious harm when the PTSD diagnosis is attached to someone whose troubles are in fact the manifestation of a different problem.

There have been debates in psychiatric circles over redefining or reshaping the concept of PTSD. While I can see the potential danger of relabeling PTSD as, for example, a "traumatic stress injury" without any firm biological science behind it, those in the non-clinical realm should nonetheless be encouraged to think of mental injuries along a spectrum, rather than to view things according to a trauma-or-nothing framework.* If we think of mental injuries in the same manner as physical ones—just as there are varying degrees of physical injuries there are also different severities of mental erosion—then perhaps we could begin to more accurately separate devastating mental injuries from

---

* There is a danger here because people can be diagnosed with things like mild traumatic brain injury—which results from exposure to things like bomb blasts—while still having clean brain scans. What, then, is an injury, and what is a disorder?

everyday stresses or setbacks. Conceptualizing things this way may help us to push back against the trauma juggernaut that has pigeon-holed numerous mental health challenges into the PTSD category.

Research shows, moreover, that those with "subthreshold PTSD"—that is, people who experience some symptoms of PTSD after a traumatic event but not enough to qualify for the diagnosis—suffer in the same manner (from distress, persistent nightmares, etc.) as those diagnosed with the disorder. Again, this should cause us to ask questions about what is really going on here. Could it be that their "subthreshold PTSD" is really something else? Are we neglecting the moral and spiritual components of being human, or the fact that we are social creatures whose thoughts and complexities cannot be easily placed in tidy categories?

Now that I understand what I've been through, I contend that I don't have PTSD. I believe instead that I have a stress injury that stems primarily from severe and repeated moral conflict. In the 1990s and early 2000s, when PTSD was still a fairly new topic of discussion in Canada, psychiatrists were unsure of what to make of sick peacekeepers that had witnessed the worst in humanity but had been unable to stop it. Like numerous others, I was thrown into the PTSD bucket, but I still don't believe that that term fully explains my condition or accurately describes what I feel. I would go even further and say that the reason many veterans do not recover from PTSD, even though they've received proper treatment and have had years of distance from their stress, is that they never had PTSD in the first place.

As my psychiatrist friend Dr. Don Richardson told me, "physicians and clinicians like things to be clean." But human nature and the myriad ways our mood, mind, and world view can be altered by external events prohibits mental phenomena from fitting into precise categories. Separating trauma from grief or stress from trauma is not always as easy as we've been led to believe. A growing number of psychiatrists, Don among them, have expressed openness about reconsidering PTSD in light of emerging research and the expansion of the PTSD diagnoses over the past several decades.

Personally, I believe we need to further explore the concept of stress injuries and the related concept of moral injuries—that is, an injury that occurs when humans are placed in situations that injure their moral conscience. As with many traumatic or severely stressful events, moral injury occurs in its most extreme form when soldiers are sent overseas on peacekeeping or combat operations. But civilians, too, can be placed in very difficult situations that don't necessarily fit into a medical rubric, but which still affect their ability to see the world in the same light as before, and which affect their daily functioning in both minor and major ways. Likewise, they can incur cumulative stress that eventually topples them without that stress necessarily being traumatic. Sometimes people just get worn down. By focusing more on the moral and spiritual components of stress and trauma, we might then begin to effectively separate distinct maladies without misusing the PTSD concept, and without convincing numerous Canadians that they need medical help when their injury may require other forms of aid.

Bringing morality into the mix would help Canadians to connect with and support one another in a communal, non-clinical manner—something that a purely medical approach to trauma denies. Perhaps most importantly, greater emphasis on the moral aspects of mental health *in general* would help us to think of our mental state in multi-dimensional terms. Not all hardships constitute trauma, and it is time we think of mental health—and mental illness—in a broader framework, one that incorporates medicine, morality, and even spirituality. I am *not* challenging the legitimacy of the PTSD concept, nor am I trying to downplay the cumulative effect that workplace and life stresses can have on a person's mental health. People impacted by cumulative stress sometimes feel so debilitated that, in their mind, the word *trauma* seems fitting. But often those feeling weighed down by life need a friendly shoulder to lean on more than a doctor. One of the first steps toward broadening our thinking is developing a robust, preventive mental health system that helps people *before* their problems become debilitating, and before they feel traumatized.

SADLY, THE MENTAL health system in Canada evolved as the poor cousin of Canadian health care. Historically, the health-care system's mental health component has been underfunded, in part because the level of knowledge about mental health issues was nowhere near that of physical illnesses, in part because of stigma, but also because it wasn't until fairly recently that the public took any interest in the subject. For a long time very few Canadians cared about what happened to those deemed "lunatics," "crazy" or "insane"; indeed, people with mental health issues were often kept in large mental hospitals, outside of public view. Treatments were usually hit or miss, and health professionals often felt uncomfortable dealing with patients with mental health problems. The siloing of medical treatment over time and the lack of understanding about the role of social support further worsened the situation.

The deinstitutionalization movement of the 1960s, which slowly emptied provincial mental hospitals throughout the next several decades, forced Canadians to notice the existence and prevalence of mental health conditions, ranging from minor anxiety to paranoid schizophrenia: the problem was far more difficult to ignore when it looked people in the face on street corners of major cities like Toronto, Vancouver, and Montreal, or indeed lived with them. Combined with mental health education campaigns spearheaded by groups like the Canadian Mental Health Association, deinstitutionalization slowly made us aware of what we'd pushed aside for so long. Fast forward to the twenty-first century, and we now know that 30 to 40 per cent of workplace disability and sick leave claims are related to mental health issues—and the number continues to grow. Evidently, the problem now attacks both our consciences and our wallets.

We're in a serious quandary. Our relatively underfunded mental health system is facing rapidly growing numbers of people suffering from depression, anxiety, fatigue, and myriad other issues. But ironically, even as these numbers continue to grow, mental health is still a taboo subject, something that is perpetuated in part by the extremely high level of confidentiality surrounding it at both the individual and institutional levels. For example, physicians often can't and won't discuss a patient's mental health, even with the patient's family, because the system forbids it. In some cases, especially when the patient's family is part of the problem, confidentiality is completely justifiable. But in a lot of others, the family is not the cause, and yet they are still kept on the outside.

This exclusion, in and of itself, may further isolate the patient from an understanding and supportive family network, thereby worsening their illness. In some cases, this lack of family support has led to suicide. Throughout my time with OSISS, I spoke with a multitude of clinicians who hid behind doctor-patient confidentiality, even when it was clear to anyone who knew the patient that their family could have a positive impact on treatment outcomes. Even when I broached the idea of asking the *patient* if they were comfortable with their physician discussing their mental health with loved ones, the doctor usually demurred. Good families—those who can support the patient between medical appointments—are often left to twist in the wind, leaving one of the patient's most valuable resources untapped. Some physicians buck this trend, of course, and they represent small islands of hope. Taking what I would deem as a common-sense approach, they find creative ways of involving spouses and families, by both educating the family about mental health and discussing how that education can be used to help improve their loved one's condition. We need more of that outside-the-box thinking.

The problem is that the system as a whole is laden with rigidity and dogma. It lacks not only innovative leadership but also strategic governance. The system, constructed in a sort of one-size-fits-all sort of manner, is still very static. As long as the situation remains this way, we will continue to focus all of our attention on greatly overstretched clinical resources at the expense of free ones—like families—that can not only help chip away at mental health stigmas, but also provide much-needed support to patients throughout their daily lives.

Psychologist Charles Figley, a leading trauma researcher since the 1970s, sees the family as a living system, one with interrelated parts that must work together, especially in times of hardship. The whole family is affected when one of its members deals with a debilitating illness; it must therefore heal as a unit. My own family, especially

Julie, was greatly affected by my illness, and this took a significant toll on them. I can only wish that we were given the chance to be educated about mental health when we needed it most. That education might have given both Julie and me the opportunity to cope with, and potentially stave off, years of hardship that helped doom our marriage and, in its place, left a lasting sense of loss.

What the system needs is shapers and disruptors, those who can make the system evolve along with the health-care needs of Canadians. Those needs are evolving under our very eyes, and the time to act is now. Many such shapers and disruptors exist out there, but there is no systematic way for them to exert strong leadership. Limited thinking and capacity at the institutional level teaches many doctors to go by the book, and those who are natural leaders are hamstrung by their inability to make decisive changes. Medical teaching is focused in tertiary care hospitals, which means most students have few opportunities for exposure to patients in the community. They are not boots-on-the-ground physicians; instead they're mired in technology and, for this reason, sometimes lack an understanding of what it means to be truly empathetic toward their patients. This myopia leaves us with a system that is *reactive* rather than *proactive*, one that rewards those who stick close to the rules rather than those who examine and change standard practice to suit Canadians' changing needs.

A growing number of studies show the benefits of leveraging families and peer supporters to help patients with all different types of mental challenges. For example, a 2013 report by the Centre for Mental Health in London, England, showed that when properly implemented, peer support workers could decrease hospital inpatient bed use, saving the health-care system money and providing patients crucial support outside of a clinical setting. I truly believe that if we allow peer support (and by extension, family support) to be embedded in our communities as a non-clinical adjunct, we'll see not only fewer relapses of serious illness and fewer workplace health claims, but also a gradual decrease in mental health stigma. A recent study on the use of a discharge model for patients in Ontario with mental health problems clearly shows that when peer supporters are part of the process, huge improvements are noted in the patient's health; more-over, hospital costs for readmission are substantially lowered. When we empower peers and families, we demonstrate that mental illness is a problem that even laypersons can mitigate.

By reaching people before they require in-patient care, and by helping the less seriously ill cope with the stress and fatigue of mod-ern life and work, we will help create a balanced and holistic system that supports mental health for all Canadians, preventing them from ever feeling alone in their struggle. Patients don't live in their doctor's office, and it's long past time that we recognize that. When I asked Don Richardson about whether, as a psychiatrist working within the medical system, he saw a value in peer support, he replied that doctors "aren't going out into the streets or to coffee shops. That's what really kind of sold me [on peer support] from the beginning." More doctors are starting to see the benefits of peer support as an adjunct to other forms of care, and it's time that Canadians everywhere were provided with the opportunity to seek it out. But the question remains: Will our mental health system be flexible enough, visionary enough, to create strategic, systemic change? Without a bit of a nudge, I don't think so.

CANADIANS NOW OPERATE in a brain-based economy. Although nu-merous peoples' day jobs still involve physical labour, a growing num-ber of us make a living using our mind. Just like carrying bags of ce-ment for eight hours will make your arms and back hurt, many people now have tired, deadened minds from staring at computer screens and constantly mulling over technical data. Sometimes the cumulative strain of such activities can give people what I call a "sprained brain."

But just as people with physical injuries don't always need to see a doctor, neither does everyone with a sprained brain. Often, rest and support is all that's required. Unfortunately, in the workplace there is usually no alternative to medical intervention. When you complain of mental health problems, chances are your manager or human resources representative will tell you to see a doctor, most likely through the company's EAP. That's what they've been trained to do—and of course it's better than nothing. Inadvertently, though, this sends many people into the formal health-care system who could otherwise benefit from pre-emptive, non-clinical care.

Social media must take part of the blame here as well. Despite being better connected than ever before, in many ways we've never been so *dis*connected from both ourselves and one another. Just step onto a train or an airplane, or watch numerous motorists illegally using their cell phone while driving, to witness this phenomenon in action. More and more, communication is now conducted solely through email and text message, while at the workplace water cooler many peoples' discussions revolve around questions like, "Did you get my email?" Even stranger, co-workers sitting just across the room from one another now often email each other rather than speak in person. Human beings are social creatures, and yet technology has in some respects become a wedge in our society's social fabric.

There are a lot of buzzwords and catchy terms thrown around in the corporate world, things like *work-life balance*, or *employee engagement*. The problem is, many companies use these terms while giving their employees company cell phones so that they can be reached at any time of day or night. Some humane and forward-thinking companies have gone against this trend by taking steps like preventing email traffic on company servers after business hours. Though this is certainly a step in the right direction, it's really just a band-aid solution: because in the name of productivity we've pushed a dehumanizing and dehumanized culture so far that, according to Toronto's Centre for Addiction and Mental Health, mental health problems are draining the Canadian economy of over $50 billion a year (and that number is growing). To put that in perspective, this represents almost 3 per cent of our country's entire gross domestic product, and it's more than twice what we spend on national defence—the single largest discretionary item in the federal budget.

We need to create workplaces that adopt a more humane approach to mental health. The first step in this direction is for employers to think long and hard about how their policies and practices impact employees. The second is adopting a non-clinical narrative, a narrative that re-humanizes the employees and teaches them that they can make a difference in their colleagues' lives. The day that we recognize the difference between a clinical problem and a series of bad weeks will be the day when we start to change the way employers, and the public at large, deal with their fellow human beings.

WE'VE COME A long way in terms of how we think about and treat mental health, particularly our ability to recognize psychological health as a determining factor in a person's overall well-being. We talk about mental health more than ever, and numerous individuals and corporations put a lot of money toward examining the problem. This is a step in the right direction, but it's too early to celebrate such minor successes, especially since they've so far failed to stave off what is still a burgeoning problem. The proof of the pudding is in the eating, after all: if our current practices had fixed the problem, we wouldn't still be facing rising mental health-care costs and more mentally unwell workers.

Some workplaces have been early adopters of Canada's National Standard on Psychological Health and Safety in the Workplace, a guide that, among other things, helps organizations promote mental health in the workplace. They should be applauded for that. Nevertheless, they do not represent the much larger number of employers that still place the bottom line far above employee health. Even worse are those employers who publicly claim to care while privately making the situation worse through dehumanizing policies and practices. The Canadian public, too, needs to recognize that mental health is something that requires year-round attention, not just during mental health awareness campaigns. Small gestures need to be followed by serious action, because talking can only take us so far.

My mission is to help re-humanize the workplace, decrease mental health stigma, and decrease the burden of mental illness through tangible measures like peer support. I want to work with like-minded people to transform how we support those going through tough times. I've seen firsthand the power of peer support—how it brought many men and women the strength and support they needed during a criti-

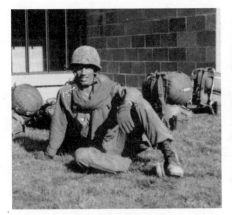 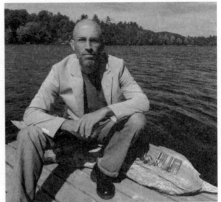

Chilliwack, B.C., spring 1984: After the final leadership exercise of my 13-week basic officer training course.

Val des Monts, Quebec, 2015: On the dock at my cottage.

cal time. I've also seen the way it can empower both sufferers of mental illness and their families, and help them to see themselves as active agents in their own recovery rather than as helpless recipients of care beyond their understanding. Canadians from all walks of life need to start treating mental health as something that requires the participation of everyone, not just professionals.

When looking back on my journey, from my time in Rwanda to the present day, my mind is still haunted by certain memories. I still think about that young girl lying on the red Rwandan soil, how her blood saturated the ground around her. That image is forever seared in my brain. But life has taken me on an interesting journey, and as cliché as it might sound, I do believe everything happens for a reason. I feel blessed that I can now serve my country in another way, by assisting organizations that want to make meaningful and lasting change. Helping them to stop talking and start walking provides me and my colleagues with rays of light as we struggle to get mental health the recognition it deserves. I look forward to the day when Canadians will view mental injuries with the same compassion and care as physical ones, and when the injured will be shouldered by friends, family, and co-workers. Then, perhaps, stories like mine will no longer have to be written.

BIBLIOGRAPHICAL NOTE

My co-author and I consulted various sources while writing this book. Readers looking to learn more about the issues explored below should consult some of the following. On the Rwandan genocide, Roméo Dallaire's memoir, *Shake Hands with the Devil: The Failure of Humanity in Rwanda,* is an excellent place to start. On the United Nations' role in various conflicts since the end of the Second World War, see Jocelyn Coulon's *Soldiers of Diplomacy: The United Nations, Peacekeeping, and the New World Order.* And for a closer look at the many challenges faced by individual soldiers in both combat and peacekeeping situations, we encourage you to seek out Carol Off's *The Ghosts of Medak Pocket: The Story of Canada's Secret War,* and Samuel Hynes's *The Soldiers' Tale: Bearing Witness to Modern War.* For an evaluation of the response of soldiers to the third-location decompression (TLD) program, see Bryan G. Garber and Mark A. Zamorski's "Evaluation of a Third-Location Decompression Program for Canadian Forces Members Returning from Afghanistan," *Military Medicine,* 177, no. 4 (2012): 397.

INDEX

Page references in *italic* indicate photographs.

ABOUT THE AUTHOR

Stéphane Grenier is a veteran of the Canadian Military who retired as a Lieutenant Colonel following twenty-nine years of service and numerous overseas missions in places such as in Cambodia, Haiti, Lebanon, and Kuwait. Most notably, he spent ten months in Rwanda in 1994/95 and six months in Kandahar, Afghanistan, in 2007.

Faced with undiagnosed PTSD upon return from Rwanda, he took a personal interest in the way the Canadian Forces was dealing with mental health issues, a mission he has now decided to broaden to the entire Canadian workforce through his work in developing non-clinical mental health interventions as a complement to traditional clinical care. In 2001 he coined the term Operational Stress Injury, and over the next decade he developed several successful and sustainable large-scale workplace mental health programs within the military.

In 2010 he was seconded to the Mental Health Commission of Canada, and since his retirement from the military in 2012, Grenier has founded a charity and created Mental Health Innovations, a social enterprise dedicated to re-humanizing workplaces in Canada. He recently launched a second company dedicated to assisting the province of Nova Scotia to enhance its mental health clinical services by leveraging peer support as a complement to traditional clinical care.

Throughout his career, Grenier has been recognized for his transformational leadership style and commended for his collaborative efforts and outstanding leadership, specifically during the post-war humanitarian disasters in Rwanda. He was awarded a Meritorious Service Cross by the Governor General of Canada for his work in the field of mental health and was recently awarded an honorary degree of Doctor of Laws by the University of Guelph.

Adam Montgomery, PhD, is an historian of medicine and Canadian military history whose current research examines the political, social, and cultural meanings of trauma over the past century. He is the author of *The Invisible Injured*, which explores how war and peacekeeping trauma affected Canadian soldiers from 1914 to 2014.